Stress, Anxiety, and Insomnia

D0779166

How You Can Benefit from Diet, Vitamins, Minerals, Herbs, Exercise, and Other Natural Methods

How to Order:

Single copies may be ordered from Prima Publishing, P.O. Box 1260BK, Rocklin, CA 95677; telephone (916) 632-4400. Quantity discounts are also available. On your letterhead, include information concerning the intended use of the books and the number of books you wish to purchase.

Stress, Anxiety, and Insomnia

How You Can Benefit from Diet, Vitamins, Minerals, Herbs, Exercise, and Other Natural Methods

Michael T. Murray, N.D.

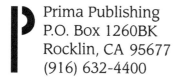
Prima Publishing
P.O. Box 1260BK
Rocklin, CA 95677
(916) 632-4400

Library of Congress Cataloging-in-Publication Data

Murray, Michael T.
  Stress, anxiety, and insomnia : how you can benefit from diet, vitamins, minerals, herbs, exercise, and other natural methods / Michael T. Murray.
    p.   cm.
  Includes bibliographical references and index.
  ISBN 1-55958-489-0
  1. Stress management.   2. Holistic medicine.   3. Anxiety—Popular works.   4. Insomnia—Popular works.   I. Title.
RA785.M87   1994
616.9'8—dc20
                                              94-36752
                                              CIP

      97 98 99 **AA** 10 9 8 7 6 5
Printed in the United States of America

Contents

4 Dietary Guidelines 27

5 Exercise and Stress Reduction 65

6 Nutritional and Herbal Support 71

SECTION *II Anxiety* 87

7 Understanding Anxiety 89

8 The Natural Approach to Anxiety 105

Lactate Levels and Anxiety 105
Flaxseed Oil and Agoraphobia 107
Another Model of Anxiety and Depression 109
Learning Optimism 121
Conditioning Your Mind and Attitude 122
Exercise to Beat Depression Naturally 124
Chapter Summary 125

9 Natural Alternatives to Anti-Anxiety Drugs 127

Kava: Nature's Herbal Anxiolytic 128
L.72 Anti-Anxiety: Natural Anxiolytic 139
GABA 140
St. John's Wort 141
Chapter Summary 142

SECTION *III* Insomnia 145

10 The Natural Approach to Insomnia 147

Preface

Stress, anxiety, and insomnia are common to many Americans. This book answers two very important questions: What causes stress, anxiety, and insomnia? What can be done to provide natural relief?

It is my hope in writing this book that more Americans will utilize the natural therapies discussed rather than filling a prescription for drugs like Prozac, Valium, Xanax, and Halcion. I believe the natural approach provides a better answer to stress, anxiety, and insomnia. The drug approach in most instances does not address the underlying cause and in many cases leads to even more problems.

When most people go to a medical doctor or psychiatrist for relief of symptoms of stress, anxiety, or insomnia, they are usually prescribed a tranquilizer or an antidepressant like Prozac. Very rarely are underlying factors or non-drug measures discussed. Natural measures are not discussed because the conventional medical doctor or psychiatrist has not been adequately educated in the role that diet, lifestyle, and attitude can play in determining an individual response to stress.

The overall influence of the pharmaceutical industry is perhaps most evident in the treatment of stress, anxiety, and insomnia. The drug companies spend huge amounts of money each year convincing doctors to emphasize drug treatment at the expense of non-drug therapies such as psychotherapy, social approaches, nutritional, herbal, or other alternative approaches.

Perhaps the biggest side effect of drug therapy is that it reinforces the practice of dealing with disease by treatment of symptoms, and diverts interest from addressing the underlying cause. However, this is not the only side effect of drug therapy, because drugs like Valium, Xanax, Prozac, and Halcion are associated with a long list of side effects including some that are very serious.

Why do physicians rely so heavily on drugs? One reason is the way they are trained. Another reason is that from the physician's perspective, it is much easier to simply write out a prescription than it is to try to figure out what psychological or physiological factors may be causing anxiety.

It is not just the physicians who are at fault here. Patients also can contribute to the problem. Many patients would much rather solve their problem by taking a pill than by taking personal responsibility for their own health.

The first step in achieving and maintaining health is taking personal responsibility. The second step is taking the appropriate action to achieve the desired results.

Achieving and maintaining health is usually quite easy if an individual follows the basic principles of health—positive mental attitude, a healthy diet, and exercise. The importance of these three essential components of a healthy lifestyle are discussed throughout this book.

Can these three essential factors be enough to eliminate stress, anxiety, and insomnia? In most cases the answer is a resounding yes. Fortunately, when additional support is needed there are a number of natural measures that have been shown to produce better results than standard drug therapy and do so without side effects.

While prescription drugs are often effective in reducing the symptoms, they have a very serious downside; they are highly addictive and can have serious side effects. Before drug treatment is used, I believe the person suffering from stress, anxiety, or insomnia should try the non-drug treatments detailed throughout this book.

Trying to "sell" people on health and the natural approach is often difficult. In order to be healthy one needs commitment. The reward is not easily seen or felt. It is usually not until the body fails us in some manner that we realize that we haven't taken care of it. Stress, anxiety, and insomnia are signs that our body and mind need support.

Regardless of the "dis-ease," the reward for most people who adopt a more positive mental attitude, eat a healthy diet, exercise regularly, and utilize natural, health promoting measures is a healthier life filled with very high levels of energy, joy, vitality, and a tremendous passion for living. That is my wish for you!

Acknowledgments

The major blessings in my life are my family and friends. My love for them truly makes life worth living.

Special appreciation goes to my wife, Gina, for being the answer to so many of my dreams; to my first child, Alexa Michelle, for being so incredibly magnificent and for teaching me so much about life; to my parents, Cliff and Patty Murray, and my grandmother, Pauline Shier, for a strong foundation and a lifetime of good memories; to Bob and Kathy Bunton for their love and acceptance; to Ben Dominitz and everyone at Prima for their commitment and support of my work; to Terry Lemerond and everyone at Enzymatic Therapy for all of their friendship and support over the years;

to Joseph Pizzorno and the students and faculty at Bastyr College who have given me encouragement and support; and finally, I am eternally grateful to all the researchers, physicians, and scientists who over the years have strived to better understand the use of natural medicines. Without their work, this series would not exist, and medical progress would halt.

Michael T. Murray, N. D.
October, 1994

Before You Read On

- Do not self-diagnose. Proper medical care is critical to good health. If you have symptoms suggestive of an illness, please consult a physician—preferably a naturopath, holistic physician or osteopath, chiropractor, or other natural health care specialist.
- If you are currently taking a prescription medication, you absolutely must consult your doctor before discontinuing it.
- If you wish to try the natural approach, discuss it with your physician. Since he or she is most likely unaware of the natural alternatives available, you may need to do some educating. Bring this book along with you to the doctor's office. The natural alternatives being recommended are based upon published studies in medical journals. Key references are provided if your physician wants additional information.
- Remember, although many natural alternatives, such as nutritional supplements and plant-based medicines, are effective on their own, they work even better if they are part of a comprehensive natural treatment plan that focuses on diet and lifestyle.

Stress

1

What Is Stress?

Most Americans know something about stress. In fact, most of us believe that everyday stress is part of modern living. Job pressures, family arguments, financial pressures, and time management are just a few of the "stressors" most of us face on a daily basis. Although we most often think of a stressor as something that causes us to feel "stressed out," technically speaking a stressor may be almost any disturbance—heat or cold, environmental toxins, toxins produced by microorganisms, physical trauma, or strong emotional reactions—that can trigger a number of biological changes to produce what is commonly known as the stress response.

Fortunately for us, control mechanisms in the body are geared toward counteracting the everyday stresses of life. Most often the stress response is so mild the work of the body goes entirely unnoticed. However, if stress is extreme, unusual, or long-lasting, these control mechanisms can be overwhelmed and the effects of stress can be quite harmful.

Recognizing Stress

Have you ever been suddenly frightened? If you have, you know what it feels like to have adrenaline surge through your body. Adrenaline is released from your adrenal glands, a pair of glands that lie on top of each kidney. Adrenaline was designed to give the body that extra energy boost to escape from danger. Unfortunately, it can also make us feel stress, anxiety, and nervousness.

Many people may not recognize what is causing them to feel stressed; all they notice are the physical signs of stress such as insomnia, depression, fatigue, headache, upset stomach, digestive disturbances, and irritability. Many people going to physicians with these complaints may be suffering from unrecognized stressors.

To determine the role that stress may play, many physicians utilize a popular method of rating stress levels, the Social Readjustment Rating Scale, developed by Holmes and Rahe (Table 1.1 on page 6).[1] The scale was originally designed to predict the likelihood of a person getting a serious disease due to stress. Various life-change events are numerically rated according to their potential for causing disease. Notice that even events commonly viewed as positive, such as an outstanding personal achievement, may carry with them significant stress.

Interpreting Your Score

The standard interpretation of the Social Readjustment Rating Scale is that a total of 200 or more units in one year is predictive of the likelihood of getting a serious disease. I also utilize the scale as an opportunity to gain insight into a person's stress level. Not everyone reacts to stressful events in the same way. I use the scale as a rough indicator of a person's stress level.

If I believe a person is under a great deal of immediate stress or has endured a fair amount of stress over a period of months or longer, I will prescribe a comprehensive stress management approach (detailed in Chapter 2).

Understanding Stress

It is important to understand the stress response. Ultimately, the success of any stress management program will depend on its ability to improve an individual's immediate and long-term response to stress.

The stress response is actually part of a larger response known as the general adaptation syndrome. To fully understand how to combat stress, it is important to take a closer look at this syndrome.

The general adaptation syndrome consists of three phases: alarm, resistance, and exhaustion.[2] These phases are largely controlled and regulated by the adrenal glands.

The General Adaptation Syndrome

The initial response to stress is the alarm reaction, often referred to as the fight or flight response. The fight or flight response is triggered by reactions in the brain that ultimately cause the pituitary gland (the master gland of the body's entire hormonal system, located at the center of the base of the brain) to release a hormone called *adrenocorticotropic hormone* (ACTH). This causes the adrenals to secrete adrenaline and other stress-related hormones.

The fight or flight response is designed to counteract danger by mobilizing the body's resources for immediate physical activity. As a result, the heart rate and force of contraction increases to provide blood to areas necessary for

Table 1.1   Social Readjustment Rating Scale

Rank	Life Event	Mean Value
1	Death of spouse	100
2	Divorce	73
3	Marital separation	65
4	Jail term	63
5	Death of a close family member	63
6	Personal injury or illness	53
7	Marriage	50
8	Fired at work	47
9	Marital reconciliation	45
10	Retirement	45
11	Change in health of family member	44
12	Pregnancy	40
13	Sex difficulties	39
14	Gain of a new family member	39
15	Business adjustment	39
16	Change in financial state	38
17	Death of a close friend	37
18	Change to different line of work	36
19	Change in number of arguments with spouse	35
20	Large mortgage	31
21	Foreclosure of mortgage or loan	30
22	Change in responsibilities at work	29
23	Son or daughter leaving home	29
24	Trouble with in-laws	29
25	Outstanding personal achievement	28
26	Wife begins or stops work	26
27	Begin or end school	26
28	Change in living conditions	25
29	Revision of personal habits	24
30	Trouble with boss	23
31	Change in work hours or conditions	20
32	Change in residence	20
33	Change in schools	20
34	Change in recreation	19
35	Change in church activities	19

Table 1.1   *(continued)*

Rank	Life Event	Mean Value
36	Change in social activities	18
37	Small mortgage	17
38	Change in sleeping habits	16
39	Change in number of family get-togethers	15
40	Change in eating habits	15
41	Vacation	13
42	Christmas	12
43	Minor violations of the law	11

response to the stressful situation. Blood is shunted away from the skin and internal organs, except the heart and lungs; at the same time the amount of blood supplying needed oxygen and glucose to the muscles and brain is increased. The rate of breathing increases to supply necessary oxygen to the heart, brain, and exercising muscle. Sweat increases to eliminate toxic compounds from the body and to lower body temperature. Production of digestive secretions is severely reduced, since digestive activity is not critical for counteracting stress. And blood sugar levels go up dramatically as the liver dumps stored glucose into the bloodstream.

While the alarm phase is usually short-lived, the next phase—the resistance reaction—allows the body to continue fighting a stressor long after the effects of the fight or flight response have worn off. Other hormones, such as cortisol and other corticosteroids secreted by the adrenal cortex, are largely responsible for the resistance reaction. For example, these hormones stimulate the conversion of protein to energy so that the body has a large supply of energy long after glucose stores are depleted and also promote the retention of sodium to keep blood pressure elevated.

Besides providing the energy and circulatory changes necessary to deal effectively with stress, the resistance reaction initiates those changes required for meeting emotional crisis, performing strenuous tasks, and fighting infection. However, while the effects of adrenal cortex hormones are quite necessary when the body is faced with danger, prolongation of the resistance reaction due to continued stress increases the risk of significant disease, including diabetes, high blood pressure, and cancer, and results in the final stage of the general adaptation syndrome, exhaustion.

Exhaustion may manifest by a total collapse of body function or a collapse of specific organs. Two major causes of exhaustion are losses of potassium ions and depletion of adrenal glucocorticoid hormones like cortisone.[1] When cells of the body lose potassium they function less effectively and eventually die. When adrenal glucocorticoid stores become depleted, hypoglycemia results and cells of the body do not receive enough glucose or other nutrients.

Another cause of exhaustion is weakening of the organs. Prolonged stress places a tremendous load on many organ systems, especially the heart, blood vessels, adrenals, and immune system.

Conditions Strongly Linked to Stress[2]

Angina

Asthma

Autoimmune disease

Cancer

Cardiovascular disease

Common cold

Diabetes (adult onset—Type II)

Depression

Headaches

Hypertension

Immune suppression
Irritable bowel syndrome
Menstrual irregularities
Premenstrual tension syndrome
Rheumatoid arthritis
Ulcerative colitis
Ulcers

Stress: A Healthy View

The father of modern stress research was Hans Selye, M.D. Having spent many years studying stress, Dr. Selye probably has the best perspective on the role of stress and disease. According to Dr. Selye, stress in itself should not be viewed in a negative context. It is not the stressor that brings on the response, but the individual's internal reaction which then triggers the response. This internal reaction is highly individualized. What one person may experience as stress, the next person may view entirely differently. Selye perhaps summarized his view best in his book *The Stress of Life*.[2]

> No one can live without experiencing some degree of stress all the time. You may think that only serious disease or intensive physical or mental injury can cause stress. This is false. Crossing a busy intersection, exposure to a draft, or even sheer joy are enough to activate the body's stress mechanisms to some extent. Stress is not even necessarily bad for you; it is also the spice of life, for any emotion, any activity causes stress. But, of course, your system must be prepared to take it. The same stress which makes one person sick can be an invigorating experience for another.

The key statement that Dr. Selye made may be, "Your system must be prepared to take it." The individual can help prepare and bolster the stress-fighting system by adopting an effective, comprehensive stress management program, as outlined in Chapter 2.

Chapter Summary

Stress is defined as any disturbance—heat or cold, chemical toxins, microorganisms, physical trauma, or strong emotional reactions—that can trigger the stress response. How an individual handles stress plays a major role in determining their level of health.

2

Comprehensive
Stress Management

To deal effectively with stress an individual must concentrate on four equally important components which are like four cornerstones or four legs on a table. Lack of attention to any of these key factors will ultimately lead to a breakdown in the bodily system, much as the breaking of a leg of a table would lead to total collapse of the table. The four cornerstones of effective stress management are: (1) techniques to calm the mind and promote a positive mental attitude; (2) a healthful diet designed to nourish the body and support physiological processes; (3) exercise; and (4) supplementary measures designed to support the body as a whole, but especially the adrenal glands.

The next four chapters detail specific methods to support these four cornerstones. The level or degree of support necessary depends on your current stress status. For example, if you scored very high on the Social Readjustment Scale, I would recommend that you employ all methods to support your body and mind's response to stress. If you feel stressed, fatigued, or "burned out," I would also recommend that you follow the program. If you do not suffer from undue high stress, you may not need the supplementary measures discussed in Chapter 6.

Negative Coping Patterns

Before considering the positive methods for dealing with stress, it is important to identify whether you are employing methods that I refer to as negative coping methods. I label them negative because they simply do not support the body and good health.

Whether you are currently aware of it or not, you already have a pattern for coping with stress. Unfortunately, most people have found patterns and methods that ultimately do not support good health. If you are going to be truly successful in coping with stress, negative coping patterns must be identified and replaced with positive ways of coping. Try to identify below any negative or destructive coping patterns you may have developed:

Dependence on chemicals
Drugs, legal or illicit
Alcohol
Smoking
Overeating
Too much television
Emotional outbursts
Feelings of helplessness
Overspending
Excessive behavior

Chemical Dependencies

The United States is a nation of addicts according to Joseph Beasley, M.D., the primary investigator involved in the famous Kellogg Report, *The Impact of Nutrition, Environment, and Lifestyle on Illness in America.* The level of addiction ranges from the responsible person who "can't get started in the morning" without a cup of coffee to the strung-out crack addict. Dr. Beasley offers some considerable evidence to support his belief.[1]

- Americans consume 450 million cups of coffee each day.
- Half of the population between the ages of 30 and 60 define themselves as coffee drinkers.
- At least 15 million Americans drink six or more cups or coffee each day.
- Of American adults, 30% smoke at least half a pack of cigarettes each day.
- At least 10% of the population is addicted to alcohol.
- Anywhere from 24% to 33% of the population consume 4 to 13 drinks daily.
- One-third of high school seniors report "binge drinking" (five or more drinks in a row) at least once in the last two weeks.
- Every year Americans swallow more than 5 billion tranquilizers like Valium and Xanax.
- Cocaine addiction afflicts at least 2.2 million persons, with about 1% of the United States population using cocaine at least once per week.

In many instances, people claim that they smoke, drink alcohol, or take drugs because it calms them. In reality, these substances complicate matters. The relaxation or chemical high these drugs induce is short-lived and ultimately adds more stress to the system. Individuals suffering from stress-related disorders (see page 8), anxiety, depression, or other psychological conditions must absolutely stop drinking coffee and other sources of caffeine, alcohol, smoking, and other destructive habits. Instead, choose health.

The Need to Get High

There appears to be an inherent need for humans to get high. Does this need to be the chemical high that most Americans seek? No. Think back to some fantastic moments in your life. Most of us have experienced an extreme natural high at least once in our lives. What was the moment in your life that seemed almost magical? Was it the first time your wife or lover said they loved you? How about the birth of your first child? Or, how about when you accomplished one of your dreams? Didn't these moments seem almost unreal? Did you feel as if you were naturally high?

All the drugs that act on the brain do so by mimicking or enhancing the activity of natural compounds already present in the brain. Within you lie all the chemicals required for every emotion you can possibly experience. The key is not to take drugs to try and duplicate these feelings, but rather to learn how to create the feelings inside of you so that you can conjure them up whenever you want. Your mind is a powerful tool. You can use your mind to create powerful positive emotions that can give you a natural high to help you better cope with stress.

Here is how. First of all, how did you feel when I asked you to recall a powerful positive experience in your life? As I was writing the last few paragraphs I was overcome by incredible feelings of love, appreciation, and energy. Why? Because as I was writing I couldn't help but recall some of the magical moments in my own life. I started looking at all the things that I am grateful for in my life. My mind naturally started thinking about all the people that I love and cherish. I found myself laughing as I remembered some of the best times of my life. What does this have to do with coping with stress? Recalling positive feelings and moments on a regular basis conditions your mind to continue to experience these emotions thus allowing you to be in a more resourceful state of mind.

All of this may sound a bit funny, but believe me it works. In the next chapter there are additional tips to help condition your brain and emotions to experience more pleasurable, less stressful moments in your life. If you suffer from anxiety, the recommendations in Chapters 8 and 9 are particularly useful, but you will also want to follow all of the general recommendations given here in Section I.

Time Management

One of the biggest stressors for most people is time. They simply do not feel they have enough of it. Time management does not mean squeezing more and more work into less and less time. It means learning to plan your time more effectively to allow more time for those activities in life that you enjoy. Here are seven tips that really seem to work!

1. *Set priorities.* Realize that you can only accomplish so much in a day. Decide what is important, and limit your efforts to that goal.

2. *Organize your day.* There are always interruptions and unplanned demands on your time, but create a definite plan for the day based on your priorities. Avoid the pitfall of always letting the "immediate demands" control your life.

3. *Delegate authority.* Delegate as much authority and work as you can. You can't do everything yourself. Learn to train and depend on others.

4. *Tackle tough jobs first.* Handle the most important tasks early, while your energy levels are high. Leave the busywork or running around for later in the day.

5. *Minimize meeting time.* Schedule meetings to bump up against the lunch hour or quitting time; that way they can't last forever.

6. *Avoid putting things off.* Work done under pressure of an unreasonable deadline often has to be redone. That creates more stress than if it had been done right the first time. Plan ahead.

7. *Don't be a perfectionist.* You can never really achieve perfection. Do your best in a reasonable amount of time, then move on to other tasks. If you find time, you can always come back later and polish the work some more.

Stress and Relationships

Other major causes of stress for many people are interpersonal relationships. Interpersonal relationships can be divided into three major categories: marital, family, and job-related. Humans are social beings. We need to relate to each other to nourish our minds and souls. However, relationships (or the lack of relationships) can be a significant source of stress.

The quality of any relationship ultimately comes down to the quality of the communication. Learning to communicate effectively goes a long way in reducing stress and occasional (or frequent) conflicts. Here are seven tips to effective communication, regardless of the type of relationship.

1. *Learn to be a good listener.* This is most important. Allow those you are communicating with to really share their feelings and thoughts—uninterrupted. Empathize with them, put yourself in their shoes. If you first seek to understand, you will find yourself being better understood.

2. *Be an active listener.* Act really interested in what the other person is telling you. Listen, instead of thinking about your response. Ask questions to gain more information or clarify what is being said. Good questions open lines of communication.

3. *Be a reflective listener.* Restate or reflect back to the other person your interpretation of what he or she is telling you. This simple technique shows the other person that you are both listening and understanding. If you have heard wrongly, this may cause short-term conflict, but it is certainly worth the risk, as you can begin to clarify each other's thoughts.

4. *Wait to speak until the person or people you want to communicate with are listening.* If they are not ready to listen, no matter how well you communicate your message will not be heard.

5. *Don't try to talk over somebody.* If you find yourself being interrupted, relax and wait. If you are courteous and allow the others to speak, eventually (unless they are extremely rude) they will respond likewise. If they don't, point out that they are interrupting the communication process. You can only do this if you have been a good listener. Double standards in relationships seldom work.

6. *Help others become active listeners.* Ask if they understood what you were communicating. Ask them to tell you what they heard. If they don't seem to understand what you are saying, keep talking until they do.

7. *Don't be afraid of long silences.* Human communication involves much more than human words. A great deal can be communicated during silences. Unfortunately, in many situations silence makes us feel uncomfortable. Relax. Some people need silence to collect their thoughts and feel safe. During silences remain an active listener.

Chapter Summary

Comprehensive stress management requires: (1) techniques to calm the mind and promote a positive mental attitude; (2) a healthful diet designed to nourish the body and support physiological processes; (3) exercise; and (4) supplementary measures designed to support the adrenal glands. In addition, two major areas of stress—time management and interpersonal relationships—must also be addressed.

Identifying and eliminating negative coping strategies and replacing them with the positive coping methods contained in this book will promote a better chance of long-term health.

3

Calming the Mind and Body

Learning to calm the mind and body is extremely important in relieving stress. When the mind and body are calm, stress seems to simply melt away. Among the easiest methods are relaxation exercises. The goal is to produce a physiological response known as the relaxation response, which is exactly the opposite of the stress response. Although an individual may relax by simply sleeping, watching television, or reading a book, relaxation techniques are designed specifically to produce the relaxation response.

Another great way to relieve stress and built-up tensions is to receive regular massage or bodywork. These relaxation techniques are like icing on the cake; nonetheless, regular massage or bodywork is encouraged as part of a comprehensive stress management program.

The Relaxation Response

The relaxation response is a term that was coined by Harvard professor and cardiologist Herbert Benson, M.D., in the early 1970s to describe a physiological response that is the opposite of the stress response.[1] With the stress response, the sympathetic nervous system dominates. With the relaxation response, the parasympathetic nervous system dominates. The parasympathetic nervous system controls bodily functions such as digestion, breathing, and heart rate during periods of rest, relaxation, visualization, meditation, and sleep. While the sympathetic nervous system is designed to protect us against immediate danger, the parasympathetic system is designed for repair, maintenance, and restoration of the body.

The Stress Response
- The heart rate and force of contraction of the heart increases to provide blood to areas necessary for response to the stressful situation.
- Blood is shunted away from the skin and internal organs, except the heart and lungs, while at the same time the amount of blood supplying needed oxygen and glucose to the muscles and brain is increased.
- The rate of breathing increases to supply necessary oxygen to the heart, brain, and exercising muscle.
- Sweat production increases to eliminate toxic compounds produced by the body and to lower body temperature.
- Production of digestive secretions is severely reduced since digestive activity is not critical for counteracting stress.
- Blood sugar levels are increased dramatically as the liver dumps stored glucose into the bloodstream.

The Relaxation Response
- The heart rate is reduced and the heart beats more effectively. Blood pressure is reduced.

- Blood is shunted towards internal organs, especially those organs involved in digestion.
- The rate of breathing decreases as oxygen demand is reduced during periods of rest.
- Sweat production decreases as a person who is calm and relaxed does not experience nervous perspiration.
- Production of digestive secretions is increased, greatly improving digestion.
- Blood sugar levels are maintained in the normal physiological range.

Achieving the Relaxation Response

To achieve the relaxation response a variety of techniques can be used. It really doesn't matter which way you choose; in the end the goal is the same physiological state—deep relaxation. You might choose meditation, prayer, progressive relaxation, self-hypnosis, or biofeedback. The best relaxation technique for each person is totally individual. The important thing is to set aside at least 5 to 10 minutes each day for focused relaxation. These sessions will also remind you to breathe throughout the day in a more relaxed, effective manner.

How to Breathe

Producing deep relaxation requires learning how to breathe. Have you ever noticed how a baby breathes? With each breath the baby's abdomen rises and falls as the baby breathes with the diaphragm, a dome-shaped muscle that separates the chest cavity from the abdominal cavity. If you are like most adults, you tend to fill only your upper chest because you do not utilize the diaphragm. Shallow breathing tends to produce tension and fatigue.

One powerful method of producing less stress and more energy in the body is to learn how to breathe with the diaphragm, which dramatically changes the body's physiology. It literally activates the relaxation centers in the brain. Here is a popular technique I use to train people to breathe with their diaphragm.

- Find a comfortable, quiet place to lie down or sit.
- Place your feet slightly apart. Place one hand on your abdomen near your navel. Place the other hand on your chest.
- You will be inhaling through your nose and exhaling through your mouth.
- Concentrate on your breathing. Note which hand is rising and falling with each breath.
- Gently exhale most of the air in your lungs.
- Inhale while slowly counting to 4. As you inhale, slightly extend your abdomen, causing it to rise about 1 inch. Make sure that you are not moving your chest or shoulders.
- As you breathe in, imagine the warm air flowing in. Imagine this warmth flowing to all parts of your body.
- Pause for 1 second, then slowly exhale to a count of 4. As you exhale, your abdomen should move inward.
- As the air flows out, imagine all your tension and stress leaving your body.
- Repeat the process until a sense of deep relaxation is achieved.

Now that you know how, remember to breathe with your diaphragm as much as possible, especially during times of increased stress.

Progressive Relaxation

Progressive relaxation is based on a very simple procedure of comparing tension against relaxation. Many people are not aware of the sensation of relaxation. In progressive relaxation an individual is taught what it feels like to relax by comparing relaxation to muscle tension.

Each muscle will first be asked to contract forcefully for a period of 1 to 2 seconds and then give way to a feeling of relaxation. If you do this progressively through all the muscles of the body, eventually a deep state of relaxation will result. The procedure begins with contracting the muscles of the face and neck, holding the contraction for a period of at least 1 to 2 seconds and then relaxing the muscles. Next the upper arms and chest are contracted then relaxed, followed by the lower arms and hands. The process is repeated progressively down the body, through the abdomen, buttocks, thighs, calves, and feet. This whole practice is repeated two or three times. This technique is often used in the treatment of anxiety and insomnia.

Progressive relaxation, deep breathing exercises, or the use of some other stress reduction technique is an important component of a comprehensive stress management program. Remember to set aside at least 5 to 10 minutes each day just to relax.

As you learn to relax, you may notice a great deal of muscular tension or stress in certain areas of your body. That is where the next phase of physical care of the body comes into play—bodywork.

Bodywork

The need to touch and be touched is universal. Around the world, bodywork practitioners are relied upon much more than in the United States. However, there is a growing popularity for bodywork treatments by Americans.

Many different types of bodywork can provide benefit in relieving stress, tension, and anxiety, including various massage techniques, chiropractic spinal adjustment and manipulation, Rolfing, reflexology, shiatsu, and many more. All of these techniques can work, so it is really a matter of personal preference. Find a technique or practitioner that you really like and incorporate bodywork into your routine.

I have experienced a broad range of bodywork, from Rolfing and deep tissue massage (often referred to as a sport massage) to more gentle techniques like craniosacral therapy and Trager massage. My experience has led me to the conclusion that the therapist is more critical to the outcome than the technique. The technique is only a tool. The result is largely dependent upon the person using the tool. That being said, my own personal belief is that deep tissue work like Rolfing and Hellerwork are probably the most powerful bodywork techniques for creating change in body posture and energy levels.

Unlike other bodywork techniques like massage and spinal adjustment which focus on the muscles and spine, Rolfing and Hellerwork focus on the elastic sheathing network that helps support the body, keeping bones, muscles, and organs in place. This network is known as the *fascia.* According to Rolfers and Hellerwork practitioners, the fascia can be damaged by physical injury, emotional trauma, and bad postural habits. The result is that the body is thrown out of alignment. Rolfing, Hellerwork, and other deep tissue treatments attempt to bring the body back into balance to restore efficiency of movement and increase mobility by stretching and lengthening the fascia to restore it to its natural form and pliability.

Rolfing or Hellerwork treatments consist of 10 or 11 sessions, each lasting between 60 and 90 minutes. Treatments are sequential, beginning with more superficial treatments and ending with deeper massage. Deep tissue treatment can be quite painful, but the rewards are worth it: improved breathing, posture, tolerance to stress, and, of course, energy levels. In addition, many people going through deep tissue therapy such as Rolfing and Hellerwork report resolution of emotional conflicts. It seems that many painful or traumatic experiences are stored in the fascia and muscles as tension.

Releasing the tension and restoring freedom in the fascia can produce remarkable increases in energy levels.

If Rolfing or Hellerwork is too painful, a light touch therapy called Tragerwork or Trager massage feels incredibly pleasurable and can produce similar, but more gradual results. Tragerwork was the innovation of Milton Trager, M.D. According to Trager, we all develop mental and physical patterns that may limit our movements or contribute to fatigue, pain, or tension. During a typical session, the practitioner gently and rhythmically rocks, cradles, and moves the client's body and encourages the client to see that freedom of movement and relaxation are entirely possible. The aim of the treatment is not so much to massage or manipulate, but rather to promote feelings of lightness, freedom, and well-being. Clients are also taught a series of exercises to do at home. Called Mentastics, these simple, dance-like movements are designed to help clients maintain and enhance the feelings of flexibility and freedom they may have experienced during the sessions.

Chapter Summary

Learning to calm the mind and body are essential goals in a comprehensive stress management program. A variety of techniques can be used to produce the relaxation response—a physiologic response that is just the opposite of the stress response. Diaphragmatic breathing relieves tensions and promotes relaxation. Regular bodywork is another great way to melt away stress and tension.

4

Dietary Guidelines

According to Hans Selye, M.D., one of the leading pioneers of stress research, the difference between stress being harmful or not is based upon the strength of the human system. What determines the strength of the human system? From a purely physiological perspective it can be strongly argued that delivery of high-quality nutrition to the cells of the body is the critical factor in determining the strength of the system.

When the eating habits of Americans are examined as a whole it is little wonder that so many people are suffering from stress, anxiety, and fatigue. Most Americans are not providing the body the nutrition it needs. When a machine does not receive the proper fuel or maintenance, how long can it be expected to run in an efficient manner? Similarly, if your body is not fed the full range of nutrients it needs, how can it be expected to stay in a state of good health?

Instead of eating foods rich in vital nutrients, most Americans consume refined foods high in calories, sugar, fat, and cholesterol. Instead of eating life-giving foods,

Americans are filling up on cheeseburgers, french fries, Twinkies, and chocolate chip cookies, and washing them down with artificially colored and flavored fruit drinks or colas. It is an undeniable fact that the three leading causes of death in the U.S. (heart disease, cancer, and strokes) are diet-related and that over one-third of our adult population is overweight.

It is estimated that each year the average American consumes 100 pounds of refined sugar and 55 pounds of fats and oils in the form of:

300 cans of soda pop

200 sticks of gum

18 pounds of candy

5 pounds of potato chips

7 pounds of corn chips, popcorn, and pretzels

63 dozen donuts and pastries

50 pounds of cakes and cookies

20 gallons of ice cream

Diet for Stress and Anxiety

This chapter details recommended dietary guidelines and discusses the role of diet in the treatment of stress and anxiety.

1. Eliminate or restrict the intake of caffeine.
2. Eliminate or restrict the intake of alcohol.
3. Eliminate refined carbohydrates from the diet.
4. Design a healthful diet.
5. Eat regular planned meals in a relaxed environment.
6. Control food allergies.

Caffeine and Stress Levels

The average American consumes 150 to 225 milligrams of caffeine daily, roughly the amount of caffeine in one to two cups of coffee. Although most people can handle this amount, some people are more sensitive to the effects of caffeine than others due to a slower elimination of these substances from the body. Even small amounts of caffeine, as found in decaffeinated coffee, is enough to affect some people adversely and produce "caffeinism," a medical condition characterized by symptoms of depression, nervousness, irritability, recurrent headache, heart palpitations, and insomnia (see Table 4.1). People prone to feeling stress and anxiety tend to be especially sensitive to caffeine.[1]

Chronic caffeine intake is linked to anxiety and depression for the same reasons that it produces mental and physical stimulation.[2] Caffeine produces significant alteration of brain chemistry. Perhaps one of the most powerful effects of caffeine is its ability to interfere with adenosine. Adenosine is kind of like the brain's own Valium. In fact, the way

Table 4.1 Caffeine Content of Coffee, Tea, and Selected Soft Drinks

Beverage	Caffeine Content (in milligrams)	Beverage	Caffeine Content (in milligrams)
Coffee (7.5-ounce cup)		*Soft drinks*	
Drip	115–150	Jolt	100
Brewed	80–35	Mountain Dew	54
Instant	40–65	Tab	47
Decaffeinated	3–4	Coca-Cola	45
		Diet Coke	45
Tea (5-ounce cup)		Dr. Pepper	40
1-min. brew	20	Pepsi Cola	38
3-min. brew	35	Diet Pepsi	36
Iced (12 ounces)	70	7 Up	0

in which Valium and similar drugs work is by mimicking the effects of adenosine in the brain. Chronic use of caffeine, by blocking adenosine as well as by altering other chemical processes in the brain, is enough to produce depression and anxiety in some people.[1]

Caffeine, at relatively small doses (50 to 200 milligrams) stimulates the brain areas associated with conscious mental processes. The result is that ideas become clearer, thoughts flow more easily, and fatigue and drowsiness decrease. Typists, for example, work faster and with fewer errors after ingesting caffeine, while drivers will notice that caffeine increases alertness and improves driving performance.[1]

However, the anti-fatigue effects of caffeine are usually only short-lived. After the initial simulation, a period of increased fatigue often results. A vicious cycle can then ensue in which a person drinks increasing amounts of caffeine to delay the onset of fatigue.[3]

Long-term use of caffeine-containing beverages, especially coffee, should be avoided in individuals suffering from stress, anxiety, insomnia, depression, or any other psychiatric disorder. The belief that caffeine provides energy is a myth: There is evidence that chronic caffeine intake may actually lead to chronic fatigue. While mice fed one dose of caffeine demonstrated significant increases in their swimming capacity, when the dose of caffeine was given for six weeks, the caffeine caused a significant decrease in swimming capacity.[4]

Several studies have found caffeine intake to be extremely high in individuals with psychiatric disorders, and the degree of fatigue they experienced was often related to how much caffeine was ingested. In one survey of a group of hospitalized psychiatric patients, 61% of those ingesting at least 750 milligrams (at least five cups of coffee) daily complained of fatigue, compared to 54% of those ingesting 250 to 749 milligrams daily, and only 24% of those ingesting less than 250 milligrams daily.[5]

Be aware that if you routinely drink coffee, abrupt cessation of coffee drinking will probably result in symptoms of caffeine withdrawal, including fatigue, headache, and an intense desire for coffee.[1,3] Fortunately, this withdrawal period doesn't last more than a day or two.

Alcohol and Stress Levels

Alcohol produces chemical stress on the body. It also increases adrenal hormone output, and interferes with normal brain chemistry and sleep cycles. While many people believe that alcohol has a calming effect, a study in 90 healthy male volunteers given either a placebo or alcohol demonstrated significant increases in anxiety scores after drinking the alcohol.[6] It is my recommendation that alcohol be avoided entirely by people with symptoms of stress, anxiety, or insomnia.

Refined Carbohydrates and Stress Levels

Refined carbohydrates (like sugar and white flour) are known to contribute to problems in blood sugar control, especially hypoglycemia (low blood sugar). When glucose levels are low (as occurs during hypoglycemia), the brain does not function properly and anxiety, dizziness, headache, clouding of vision, blunted mental acuity, emotional instability, confusion, and abnormal behavior may occur.

The association between hypoglycemia and impaired mental function is well known. Unfortunately, most individuals experiencing depression, anxiety, or other psychological conditions are rarely tested for hypoglycemia, nor are they prescribed a diet restricting refined carbohydrates.

Numerous studies in depressed individuals have shown a high percentage of hypoglycemia.[7,8] As depression is one of the most frequent causes of anxiety, this provides a link between hypoglycemia and feelings of stress. Simply eliminating refined carbohydrates from the diet is occasionally all that is needed for effective therapy in patients that have depression or anxiety due to hypoglycemia.

Diagnosing Hypoglycemia   The standard method of diagnosing hypoglycemia is the oral glucose tolerance test (GTT). However, many of the symptoms attributed to hypoglycemia may not be due to low blood sugar levels, but rather by either insulin or adrenaline. When all is considered, the most useful measure of diagnosing hypoglycemia remains assessing symptoms. The questionnaire (Figure 4.1) is an excellent screening method for hypoglycemia.

No = 0   Mild = 1   Moderate = 2   Severe = 3

Crave sweets   0   1   2   3

Irritable if a meal is missed   0   1   2   3

Feel tired or weak if a meal is missed   0   1   2   3

Dizziness when standing suddenly   0   1   2   3

Frequent headaches   0   1   2   3

Poor memory (forgetful) or concentration   0   1   2   3

Feel tired an hour or so after eating   0   1   2   3

Heart palpitations   0   1   2   3

Feel shaky at times   0   1   2   3

Afternoon fatigue   0   1   2   3

Vision blurs on occasion   0   1   2   3

Depression or mood swings   0   1   2   3

Overweight   0   1   2   3

Frequently anxious or nervous   0   1   2   3

Total: _____

Scoring:

Less than 5 = Hypoglycemia is not likely a factor

6–15 = Hypoglycemia is a likely factor

Greater than 15 = Hypoglycemia is extremely likely

Figure 4.1   Hypoglycemia questionnaire

The Glycemic Index   The "glycemic index" (Table 4.2) was developed by David Jenkins in 1981 to express the rise of blood glucose after eating a particular food.[9] The standard value of 100 is based on the rise seen with the ingestion of glucose. The glycemic index ranges from about 20 for fructose and whole barley to about 98 for a baked potato. The insulin response to carbohydrate-containing foods is similar to the rise in blood sugar.

The glycemic index is used as a guideline for dietary recommendations for people with hypoglycemia or diabetes. Basically, it is recommended to people with blood sugar problems that they avoid foods with high values and choose carbohydrate-containing foods with lower values. However, the glycemic index should not be the only dietary

Table 4.2   Glycemic Index of Some Common Foods[10]

Sugars		Grains	
Glucose	100	Bran cereal	51
Maltose	105	Bread, white	69
Honey	75	Bread, whole grain	72
Sucrose	60	Corn	59
Fructose	20	Corn flakes	80
Fruits		Oatmeal	49
Apples	39	Pasta	45
Bananas	62	Rice	70
Oranges	40	Rice, puffed	95
Orange juice	46	Wheat cereal	67
Raisins	64	*Legumes*	
Vegetables		Beans	31
Beets	64	Lentils	29
Carrot, raw	31	Peas	39
Carrot, cooked	36	*Other foods*	
Potato, baked	98	Ice cream	36
Potato (new), boiled	70	Milk	34
		Nuts	13
		Sausages	28

guideline. For example, highfat foods like ice cream and sausage have a low glycemic index because a diet high in fat has been shown to impair glucose tolerance, but these foods are still not good food choices for people with hypoglycemia or diabetes.

Designing a Healthful Diet

Most people give very little thought to the design of their diet. They are motivated to eat foods based on sensual needs rather than what their body requires. Health is largely a conscious decision. Awareness of what to eat, in what quantities, and healthy ways to prepare food is critical.

The American Dietetic Association (ADA) in conjunction with the American Diabetes Association and other groups, have developed the Exchange System, a convenient tool for the rapid estimation of the calorie, protein, fat, and carbohydrate content of a diet. Originally designed for use in designing dietary recommendations for diabetics, the exchange method is now used in the calculation and design of virtually all therapeutic diets. The ADA exchange plan does not place a strong-enough focus on the quality of food choices.

The Healthy Exchange System presented here is a healthier version because it emphasizes healthier food choices and focuses on unprocessed, whole foods. The diet is prescribed by allotting the number of exchanges (servings) allowed per food group for one day. There are seven exchange groups (lists); however, the milk and meat lists should be considered optional.

The Healthy Exchange System
List 1 Vegetables
List 2 Fruits
List 3 Breads, cereals, and starchy vegetables
List 4 Legumes

List 5 Fats

List 6 Milk

List 7 Meats, fish, cheese, and eggs

Because all food portions within each exchange list provide approximately the same calories, proteins, fats, and carbohydrates per serving, it is easy to construct a diet which has the following components:

Carbohydrates	65% to 75% of total calories
Fats	15% to 25% of total calories
Protein	10% to 15% of total calories
Dietary fiber	at least 50 grams

Of the carbohydrates ingested, 90% should be complex carbohydrates or naturally occurring sugars. Intake of refined carbohydrate and concentrated sugars (including honey, pasteurized fruit juices, and dried fruit, as well as sugar and white flour) should be limited to less than 10% of the total calorie intake.

Constructing a diet that meets these recommendations is simple using the exchange lists. In addition, the recommendations ensure a high intake of vital whole foods, particularly vegetables, rich in nutritional value. Table 4.3 shows the fat, carbohydrate, and protein composition per serving for each exchange list.

How Many Calories Do You Need?

In determining calorie needs, it is necessary to first determine ideal body weight. The most popular height and weight charts are the tables of "desirable weight" provided by the Metropolitan Life Insurance Company (Table 4.4). The most recent edition of these tables, published in 1983, gives weight ranges for men and women at one-inch increments of height for three body frame sizes.

Table 4.3   Macro-Nutrient Composition per Serving

List	Protein*	Fat	Carbohydrates	Fiber	Calories
Vegetables	3	0	11	1–3	50
Fruits	0	0	20	1–3	80
Breads, etc.	2	0	15	1–4	70
Legumes	7	0.5	15	6–7	90
Fats	0	5	0	0	45
Milk	8	0	12	0	80
Meats, etc.	7	3	0	0	55

* Quantities listed are in grams.

Table 4.4   1983 Metropolitan Height and Weight Table*

Height	Small Frame	Medium Frame	Large Frame
Men			
5'2"	128–134	131–141	138–150
5'3"	130–136	133–143	140–153
5'4"	132–138	135–145	142–156
5'5"	134–140	137–148	144–160
5'6"	136–142	139–151	146–164
5'7"	138–145	142–154	149–168
5'8"	140–148	145–157	152–172
5'9"	142–151	148–160	155–176
5'10"	144–154	151–163	158–180
5'11"	146–157	154–166	161–184
6'0"	149–160	157–170	164–188
6'1"	152–164	160–174	168–192
6'2"	155–168	164–178	172–197
6'3"	158–172	167–182	176–202
6'4"	162–176	171–187	181–207
Women			
4'10"	102–111	109–121	118–131
4'11"	103–113	111–123	120–134
5'0"	104–115	113–126	122–137
5'1"	106–118	115–129	125–140
5'2"	108–121	118–132	128–143
5'3"	111–124	121–135	131–147

Table 4.4 *(continued)*

Height	Small Frame	Medium Frame	Large Frame
5'4"	114–127	124–138	134–151
5'5"	117–130	127–141	137–155
5'6"	120–133	130–144	140–159
5'7"	123–136	133–147	143–163
5'8"	126–139	136–150	146–167
5'9"	129–142	139–153	149–170
5'10"	132–145	142–156	152–173
5'11"	135–148	145–159	155–176
6'0"	138–151	148–162	158–179

* Weights for adults age 25 to 59 years based on lowest mortality. Weight in pounds according to frame size in indoor clothing (5 pounds for men and 3 pounds for women) wearing shoes with one-inch heels.

Determining Frame Size

To make a simple determination of your frame size: Extend your arm and bend the forearm upwards at a 90 degree angle. Keep the fingers straight and turn the inside of your wrist away from your body. Place the thumb and index finger of your other hand on the two prominent bones on either side of your elbow. Measure the space between your fingers with a tape measure. Compare the measurement with the following chart for medium-framed individuals. A lower reading indicates a small frame; higher readings indicate a large frame.

Men

Height in 1" heels	Elbow breadth
5'2" to 5'3"	2½" to 2⅞"
5'4" to 5'7"	2⅝" to 2⅞"
5'8" to 5'11"	2¾" to 3"
6'0" to 6'3"	2¾" to 3⅛"
6'4"	2⅞" to 3¼"

Women

Height in 1" heels	Elbow breadth
4'10" to 5'3"	2¼" to 2½"
5'4" to 5'11"	2⅜" to 2⅝"
6'0"	2½" to 2¾"

After determining your desirable weight in pounds, convert it to kilograms by dividing it by 2.2. Next, take this number and multiply it by the following calories, depending upon activity level:

Little physical activity:	30 calories
Light physical activity:	35 calories
Moderate physical activity:	40 calories
Heavy physical activity:	45 calories

	Number of calories for	Approximate daily calorie
Weight (in kg) ×	activity level =	requirements
_____ ×	_____ =	_____ calories

Examples of Exchange Recommendations

1,500-Calorie Vegan Diet (daily intake):

List 1 (vegetables)	5 servings
List 2 (fruits)	2 servings
List 3 (breads, cereals, and starchy vegetables)	9 servings
List 4 (legumes)	2.5 servings
List 5 (fats)	4 servings

This recommendation would result in an intake of approximately 1,500 calories, of which 67% are derived from complex carbohydrates and naturally occurring sugars, 18%

from fat, and 15% from protein. The protein intake is entirely from plant sources, but still provides approximately 55 grams. This number is well above the recommended daily allowance of protein intake for someone requiring 1,500 calories. At least one-half of the fat servings should be from nuts, seeds, and other whole foods from the Fat Exchange List. The dietary fiber intake would be approximately 31 to 74.5 grams.

> Percentage of calories as carbohydrates: 67%
> Percentage of calories as fats: 18%
> Percentage of calories as protein: 15%
> Protein content: 55 grams
> Dietary fiber content: 31 to 74.5 grams

1,500-Calorie Omnivore Diet (daily intake):

List 1 (vegetables)	5 servings
List 2 (fruits)	2.5 servings
List 3 (breads, cereals, and starchy vegetables)	6 servings
List 4 (legumes)	1 serving
List 5 (fats)	5 servings
List 6 (milk)	1 serving
List 7 (meats, fish, cheese, and eggs)	2 servings

> Percentage of calories as carbohydrates: 67%
> Percentage of calories as fats: 18%
> Percentage of calories as protein: 15%
> Protein content: 61 grams (75% from plant sources)
> Dietary fiber content: 19.5 to 53.5 grams

2,000-Calorie Vegan Diet (daily intake):

List 1 (vegetables)	5.5 servings
List 2 (fruits)	2 servings

List 3 (breads, cereals, and starchy vegetables)	11 servings
List 4 (legumes)	5 servings
List 5 (fats)	8 servings

Percentage of calories as carbohydrates: 67%
Percentage of calories as fats: 18%
Percentage of calories as protein: 15%
Protein content: 79 grams
Dietary fiber content: 48.5 to 101.5 grams

2,000-Calorie Omnivore Diet (daily intake):

List 1 (vegetables)	5 servings
List 2 (fruits)	2.5 servings
List 3 (breads, cereals, and starchy vegetables)	13 servings
List 4 (legumes)	2 servings
List 5 (fats)	7 servings
List 6 (milk)	1 serving
List 7 (meats, fish, cheese, and eggs)	2 servings

Percentage of calories as carbohydrates: 66%
Percentage of calories as fats: 19%
Percentage of calories as protein: 15%
Protein content: 78 grams (72% from plant sources)
Dietary fiber content: 32.5 to 88.5 grams

2,500-Calorie Vegan Diet (daily intake):

List 1 (vegetables)	8 servings
List 2 (fruits)	3 servings
List 3 (breads, cereals, and starchy vegetables)	17 servings
List 4 (legumes)	5 servings

List 5 (fats)   8 servings
   Percentage of calories as carbohydrates: 69%
   Percentage of calories as fats: 15%
   Percentage of calories as protein: 16%
   Protein content: 101 grams
   Dietary fiber content: 33 to 121 grams

2,500-Calorie Omnivore Diet (daily intake):

List 1 (vegetables)	8 servings
List 2 (fruits)	3.5 servings
List 3 (breads, cereals, and starchy vegetables)	17 servings
List 4 (legumes)	2 servings
List 5 (fats)	8 servings
List 6 (milk)	1 serving
List 7 (meats, fish, cheese, and eggs)	3 servings

   Percentage of calories as carbohydrates: 66%
   Percentage of calories as fats: 18%
   Percentage of calories as protein: 16%
   Protein content: 102 grams (80% from plant sources)
   Dietary fiber content: 40.5 to 116.5 grams

3,000-Calorie Vegan Diet (daily intake):

List 1 (vegetables)	10 servings
List 2 (fruits)	4 servings
List 3 (breads, cereals, and starchy vegetables)	17 servings
List 4 (legumes)	6 servings
List 5 (fats)	10 servings

   Percentage of calories as carbohydrates: 70%
   Percentage of calories as fats: 16%

Percentage of calories as protein: 14%

Protein content: 116 grams

Dietary fiber content: 50 to 84 grams

3,000-Calorie Omnivore Diet (daily intake):

List 1 (vegetables)	10 servings
List 2 (fruits)	3 servings
List 3 (breads, cereals, and starchy vegetables)	20 servings
List 4 (legumes)	2 servings
List 5 (fats)	10 servings
List 6 (milk)	1 serving
List 7 (meats, fish, cheese, and eggs)	3 servings

Percentage of calories as carbohydrates: 67%

Percentage of calories as fats: 18%

Percentage of calories as protein: 15%

Protein content: 116 grams (81% from plant sources)

Dietary fiber content: 45 to 133 grams

Note: Use these recommendations as the basis for calculating other calorie diets. For example, for a 4,000-calorie diet add the 2,500 to the 1,500. For a 1,000-calorie diet divide the 2,000 calorie diet in half.

The Healthy Exchange Lists

List 1: Vegetables

Vegetables are excellent sources of vitamins, minerals, and health-promoting fiber compounds. Vegetables are fantastic "diet" foods as they are very high in nutritional value but low in calories. Please notice that starchy vegetables like potatoes and yams are included in List 3: Breads, Cereals, and Starchy Vegetables. In addition to eating vegetables whole, vegetables can be consumed as fresh juice. There is also a list of "free" vegetables. These vegetables are termed "free foods" and can be eaten in any desired amount because the calories they contain are offset by the number of calories your body burns in the process of digestion. These foods are especially valuable diet foods as they help to keep you feeling satisfied between meals.

As the recommendations for vegetables in the Healthy Exchange System is quite high, many individuals may find it easier to juice their fresh, raw vegetables. Juicing allows for easy absorption of the health-giving properties of vegetables in larger amounts.

This list shows the vegetables to use for 1 vegetable serving. One cup cooked vegetables or fresh vegetable juice, and 2 cups raw vegetables equals 1 exchange:

> Artichoke (1 medium)
> Asparagus
> Bean sprouts
> Beets
> Broccoli
> Brussels sprouts
> Carrots
> Cauliflower
> Eggplant
> Greens:
>> Beet
>> Chard
>> Collard
>> Dandelion
>> Kale
>> Mustard

Spinach
Turnip
Mushrooms
Okra
Onions
Rhubarb
Rutabaga
Sauerkraut
String beans, green or yellow
Summer squash
Tomatoes, tomato juice, vegetable juice cocktail
Zucchini

The following vegetables may be used as often as desired, especially in their raw form:

Alfalfa sprouts
Bell peppers
Bok choy
Cabbage
Chicory
Celery
Chinese cabbage
Cucumber
Endive
Escarole
Lettuce
Parsley
Radishes
Spinach
Turnips
Watercress

List 2: Fruits

Fruits make excellent snacks. They contain fructose or fruit sugar, which is absorbed slowly into the bloodstream allowing the body time to utilize it. Fruits are excellent sources of vitamins and minerals as well as health-promoting fiber compounds and flavonoids. Fruits are not as nutrient-dense as vegetables because they are typically higher in calories. That is why vegetables are favored over fruits in weight-loss plans and overall healthy diets.

Fresh fruit and fruit-based items
Each of the following equals 1 serving:

Fresh juice, 1 cup (8 ounces)
Pasteurized juice, ⅔ cup
Apple, 1 large
Applesauce (unsweetened), 1 cup
Apricots, fresh, 4 medium
Apricots, dried, 8 halves
Banana, 1 medium
Berries
    Blackberries, 1 cup
    Blueberries, 1 cup
    Cranberries, 1 cup
    Raspberries, 1 cup
    Strawberries, 1½ cups
Cherries, 20 large
Dates, 4
Figs, fresh, 2
Figs, dried, 2
Grapefruit, 1
Grapes, 20

Mango, 1 small
Melons
    Cantaloupe, ½ small
    Honeydew, ¼ medium
    Watermelon, 2 cups
Nectarine, 2 small
Orange, 1 large
Papaya, 1½ cups
Peach, 2 medium
Persimmon, native, 2 medium
Pineapple, 1 cup
Plums, 4 medium
Prunes, 4 medium
Prune juice, ½ cup
Raisins, 4 tablespoons
Tangerine, 2 medium

Processed fruit and other products
Eat no more than 1 serving per day.

Honey, 1 tablespoon
Jams, jellies, preserves, 1 tablespoon
Sugar, 1 tablespoon

List 3: Breads, Cereals, and Starchy Vegetables

Breads, cereals, and starchy vegetables are classified as complex carbohydrates. Chemically complex carbohydrates are made up of long chains of simple carbohydrates or sugars. The body has to digest or break down the large sugar chains into simple sugars. Therefore, the sugar from complex carbohydrates enters the bloodstream more slowly. As a result, blood sugar levels and appetite are better controlled.

Complex carbohydrate foods like breads, cereals, and starchy vegetables are higher in fiber and nutrients but lower in calories than foods high in simple sugars like cakes and candies.

Breads, Cereals, and Starchy Vegetables
Each of the following equals 1 serving:

Breads
> Bagel, small, ½
> Dinner roll, 1
> Dried bread crumbs, 3 tablespoons
> English muffin, small, ½
> Tortilla (6-inch), 1
> Whole wheat, rye or pumpernickel, 1 slice

Cereals
> Bran flakes, ½ cup
> Cornmeal (dry), 2 tablespoons
> Cereal (cooked), ½ cup
> Flour, 2½ tablespoons
> Grits (cooked), ½ cup
> Pasta (cooked), ½ cup
> Puffed cereal (unsweetened), 1 cup
> Rice or barley (cooked), ½ cup
> Wheat germ, ¼ cup
> Other unsweetened cereal, ¾ cup

Crackers
> Arrowroot, 3
> Graham (2½-inch square), 2
> Matzo (4 by 6 inches), ½
> Rye wafers (2 by 3½ inches), 3
> Saltines, 6

Starchy vegetables
    Corn, ⅓ cup
    Corn on cob, 1 small
    Parsnips, ⅓ cup
    Potato, mashed, ½ cup
    Potato, white, 1 small
    Squash, winter, acorn, or butternut, ½ cup
    Yam or sweet potato, ¼ cup
Prepared foods
    Biscuit, 2" diameter (omit 1 fat serving), 1
    Corn bread, 2 by 2 by 1 inch (omit 1 fat serving) 1
    French fries, 2 to 3 inches long (omit 1 fat serving), 8
    Muffin, small (omit 1 fat serving), 1
    Potato or corn chips (omit 2 fat servings), 15
    Pancake, 5 by ½ inch (omit 1 fat serving), 1
    Waffle, 5 by ½ inch (omit 1 fat serving), 1

List 4: *Legumes*

Legumes are fantastic foods as they are rich in important nutrients and health-promoting compounds. Legumes help improve liver function, lower cholesterol levels, and are extremely effective in improving blood sugar control. Since obesity and diabetes have been linked to loss of blood sugar control (insulin insensitivity), legumes appear to be extremely important in weight loss plans and in the dietary management of diabetes.

Legumes
In this list, ½ cup of each item, cooked or sprouted, equals 1 serving:

Black-eyed peas
Chickpeas

Garbanzo beans
Kidney beans
Lentils
Lima beans
Pinto beans
Soybeans, including tofu (omit 1 fat serving)
Split peas
Other dried beans and peas

List 5: Fats and Oils

Animal fats are typically solid at room temperature and are referred to as saturated fats, while vegetable fats are liquid at room temperature and are referred to as unsaturated fats or oils. Vegetable oils provide the greatest source of the essential fatty acids linoleic acid and linolenic acid. These fatty acids function in our bodies as components of nerve cells, cellular membranes, and hormone-like substances. Fats also provide the body with energy.

While fats are important to human health, too much fat in the diet, especially saturated fat, is linked to numerous cancers, heart disease, and strokes. It is strongly recommended by most nutritional experts that the total fat intake be kept below 30% of the total calories. It is also recommended that at least twice as much unsaturated fats be consumed as saturated fats.

Fats and Oils
Each of the following equals 1 serving:

Mono-unsaturated
Olive oil, 1 teaspoon
Olives, 5 small

Polyunsaturated

Almonds, 10 whole

Avocado (4-inch diameter), ⅛ fruit

Peanut butter, 2 tablespoons

Peanuts

    Spanish, 20 whole

    Virginia, 10 whole

Pecans, 2 large

Seeds

    Flax, 1 tablespoon

    Pumpkin, 1 tablespoon

    Sesame, 1 tablespoon

    Sunflower, 1 tablespoon

Vegetable oil

    Canola, 1 teaspoon

    Corn, 1 teaspoon

    Flaxseed, 1 teaspoon

    Safflower, 1 teaspoon

    Soy, 1 teaspoon

    Sunflower, 1 teaspoon

Walnuts, 6 small

Saturated (use sparingly)

Butter, 1 teaspoon

Bacon, 1 slice

Cream, light or sour, 2 tablespoons

Cream, heavy, 1 tablespoon

Cream cheese, 1 tablespoon

Salad dressings, 2 teaspoons

Mayonnaise, 1 teaspoon

List 6: Milk

Is milk for everybody? Definitely not. Many people are allergic to milk or lack the enzymes necessary to digest milk. The drinking of cow's milk is a relatively new dietary practice for humans. This recent introduction of cow's milk into the human diet may be the reason so many people have difficulty with milk. Certainly milk consumption should be limited to no more than 2 servings per day.

Milk

For each of the following items, 1 cup equals 1 "milk" serving, but for some items you must omit 1 or more fat servings to maintain the nutrition balance of your diet.

Nonfat milk or yogurt

2% milk (omit 1 fat serving)

Lowfat yogurt (omit 1 fat serving)

Whole milk (omit 2 fat servings)

Yogurt (omit 2 fat servings)

List 7: Meats, Fish, Cheese, and Eggs

When choosing from this list, choose primarily from the lowfat group and remove the skin of poultry. This practice will keep the amount of saturated fat low. Although many people advocate vegetarianism, List 7 provides high concentrations of certain nutrients difficult to get in an entirely vegetarian diet, such as the full-range of amino acids, vitamin B12, and iron. Nonetheless, if you have any inflammatory condition, it is best to avoid the meat food group (with the exception of cold-water fish).

Meats, Fish, Cheese, and Eggs

Each of the following items equals 1 serving:

Lowfat items (less than 15% fat content)

Beef, 1 ounce

Baby beef, chipped beef, chuck, steak, (flank, plate), tenderloin plate ribs, round, (bottom, top), all cuts rump, spare ribs, tripe

Cottage cheese, lowfat, ¼ cup

Fish, 1 ounce

Lamb, 1 ounce

Leg, rib, sirloin, loin (roast and chops), shank, shoulder

Poultry (chicken or turkey without skin), 1 ounce

Veal, 1 ounce

Leg, loin, rib, shank, shoulder, cutlet

Medium-fat items

For each of the following items, omit ½ fat serving.

Beef, 1 ounce

Ground (15% fat), canned corned beef, rib eye, round (ground commercial)

Cheese, 1 ounce

Mozzarella, ricotta, farmer, Parmesan

Eggs, 1

Organ meats, 1 ounce

Pork, 1 ounce

Loin (all tenderloin), picnic, boiled ham, shoulder, Boston butt, Canadian bacon

Highfat items

For each of the following items, omit 2 fat servings:

Beef, 1 ounce

Brisket, corned beef, ground beef (more than 20% fat), hamburger, roasts (rib), steaks (club and rib)

Cheese, cheddar, 1 ounce

Duck or goose, 1 ounce

Lamb breast, 1 ounce

Pork, 1 ounce

    Spareribs, loin, ground pork, country-style ham, deviled ham

Menu Planning

The Healthy Exchange Lists were created to ensure that you are consuming a healthy diet that is providing adequate levels of nutrients in their proper ratio. Once you have determined your caloric needs and have calculated the number of servings you require from each Healthy Exchange List, construct a daily menu plan and follow it.

Breakfast

Breakfast is an absolute must. Healthy breakfast choices include whole grain cereals, muffins, and breads along with fresh whole fruit or fresh fruit juice. Cereals, both hot and cold, preferably from whole grains, may be the best food choices for breakfast. The complex carbohydrates in the grains provide sustained energy, and an evaluation of data from the National Health and Nutrition Examination Survey II (a national survey of the nutritional and health practices of Americans) disclosed that serum cholesterol levels are lowest among adults eating whole grain cereal for breakfast. Individuals who consumed other breakfast foods had high blood cholesterol levels, and levels were highest among those who typically skipped breakfast.

Lunch

Lunch is a great time to enjoy a nourishing bowl of soup, a large salad, and some whole grain bread. Bean soups and other legume dishes are especially good lunch selections for people with diabetes and blood sugar problems, and because of their ability to improve blood sugar regulation, bean soups are filling, yet low in calories.

Snacks

The best snacks are nuts, seeds, and fresh fruit and vegetables (including fresh fruit and vegetable juices).

Dinner

For dinner, the healthiest meals contain a fresh vegetable salad, a cooked vegetable side dish or a bowl of soup, whole grains, and legumes. The whole grains may be provided in bread, pasta, as a side dish, or part of a recipe for an entree. Legumes can be utilized in soups, salads, and main dishes.

Although a varied diet rich in whole grains, vegetables, and legumes can provide optimal levels of protein, many people like to eat meat. The important thing is not to overconsume animal products. Limit your intake to no more than 4 to 6 ounces per day and choose fish, skinless poultry, and lean cuts rather than fatty meats.

Food Allergies

In addition to following the guidelines of the Healthy Exchange System, people with symptoms of anxiety or chronic fatigue need to be concerned about food allergies. As far back as 1930, noted allergist Dr. Albert Rowe began noticing that anxiety and fatigue were key features of food allergies.[11] Originally, Dr. Rowe described a syndrome known as allergic toxemia to describe a syndrome that included the symptoms of fatigue, anxiety, muscle and joint aches, drowsiness, difficulty in concentration, and depression.

Around the 1950s, this syndrome began to be referred to as the allergic tension-fatigue syndrome.[12] With the current prevalence of the new chronic fatigue syndrome many physicians and other people are forgetting that food allergies can lead to chronic fatigue as well as anxiety.

A food allergy occurs when there is an adverse reaction to the ingestion of a food, and it may or may not be mediated by the immune system. The reaction may be caused by a food protein, starch, or other food component, or by a contaminant found in the food (colorings, preservatives, or other artificial flavorings). Other words often used to refer to a food allergy include food hypersensitivity, food anaphylaxis, food idiosyncrasy, food intolerance, pharmacologic (drug-like) reaction to food, metabolic reaction to food, and food sensitivity.

Food allergies have been implicated as a causative factor in a wide range of conditions; no part of the human body is immune from being a target cell or organ. The actual symptoms produced during an allergic response depend on the location of the immune system activation, the mediators of inflammation involved, and the sensitivity of the tissues to specific mediators. As Table 4.5 indicates, food allergies have been linked to many common symptoms and health conditions.

The number of people suffering from food allergies has increased dramatically during the last 15 years. Some physicians claim that food allergies are the leading cause of most undiagnosed symptoms and that at least 60% of the American population suffers from symptoms associated with food reactions.[13] Theories of why the incidence has increased include: increased stresses on the immune system (such as greater chemical pollution in the air, water, and food), earlier weaning and earlier introduction of solid foods to infants, genetic manipulation of plants resulting in food components with greater allergenic tendencies, and increased ingestion of fewer foods. Probably all of these and

Table 4.5 Symptoms and Diseases Commonly Associated with Food Allergy

System	Symptoms and Diseases
Gastrointestinal	Canker sores, celiac disease, chronic diarrhea, stomach ulcer, gas, gastritis, irritable colon, malabsorption, ulcerative colitis
Genitourinary	Bed-wetting, chronic bladder infections, kidney disease
Immune	Chronic infections, frequent ear infections
Mental/Emotional	Anxiety, depression, hyperactivity, inability to concentrate, insomnia, irritability, mental confusion, personality change, seizures
Musculoskeletal	Bursitis, joint pain, low back pain
Respiratory	Asthma, chronic bronchitis, wheezing
Skin	Acne, eczema, hives, itching, skin rash
Miscellaneous	Arrhythmia, edema, fainting, fatigue, headache, hypoglycemia, itchy nose or throat, migraines, sinusitis

more have contributed to the increased frequency and severity of symptoms.

Food allergies, as well as respiratory tract allergies, are also characterized by the following signs:

Dark circles under the eyes (allergic shiners)

Puffiness under the eyes

Horizontal creases in the lower lid

Chronic noncyclic fluid retention

Chronic swollen glands

Diagnosing Food Allergies   Two basic categories of tests are commonly used to diagnose food allergies: (1) food challenge and (2) laboratory methods. Each has its advantages. Food challenge methods require no additional expense, but a great deal of motivation. Laboratory procedures, such as blood tests, can provide immediate identification of suspected allergens, but are more expensive.

Elimination Diet Food Challenge

Many physicians believe that the oral food challenge is the best way to diagnose food sensitivities. There are two broad categories of food challenge testing: (1) an elimination (also known as oligoantigenic) diet, followed by food reintroduction, and (2) a pure water fast, followed by the food challenge. A note of caution: Food challenge testing should *not* be used in people with symptoms that are potentially life-threatening (such as airway constriction or severe allergic reactions).

In the elimination diet method the person is placed on a limited diet; commonly eaten foods are eliminated and replaced with either hypoallergenic foods rarely eaten, or special hypoallergenic formulas. The fewer the allergic foods, the greater the ease of establishing a diagnosis. The standard elimination diet consists of lamb, chicken, potatoes, rice, banana, apple, and a cabbage family vegetable (cabbage, Brussels sprouts, or broccoli). Variations of the elimination diet may be suitable; however, it is extremely important that no allergic foods be consumed.

The person stays on this limited diet for at least one week, up to one month. If the symptoms are related to food sensitivity, they will typically disappear by the fifth or sixth day of the diet. If the symptoms do not disappear it is possible that a reaction to a food in the elimination diet is responsible; in that case try an even more restricted diet.

After one week, reintroduce individual foods according to some plan where the patient begins eating a particular food every two days. Methods range from reintroducing only a single food every two days, to one every one or two meals. Usually after the one-week "cleansing" period, the patient will develop an increased sensitivity to offending foods.

Reintroduction of sensitive foods will typically produce a more severe or recognizable symptom than before. Maintain a careful, detailed record, describing when foods were reintroduced and what symptoms appeared at that time. It can be very useful to track the wrist pulse during reintroduction, as pulse changes may occur when an allergic food is consumed.

For many people, elimination diets offer the most effective means of detection. Because one can sometimes dramatically experience the effects of food reactions, motivation to eliminate the food can be high. The downside of this procedure is that it is time consuming and requires discipline and motivation.

Laboratory Methods to Diagnose Food Allergies

The skin prick test (or skin scratch test) commonly employed by many allergists only tests for allergies mediated by a particular antibody known as IgE. As only about 10% to 15% of all food allergies are mediated by IgE, this test is of little value in diagnosing most food allergies. In the skin prick test, food extracts are placed on the patient's skin using a scratch or prick method. If the patient is allergic to the food, a welt will form immediately as the allergen reacts with IgE-sensitized cells in the patient's skin.

A better route to follow in the laboratory diagnosis of food allergies is the use of special blood tests. The blood tests are extremely convenient and relatively accurate. The downside is that they also tend to be expensive (around $200 for a full panel). The RAST (radio-allergo-sorbent test) and the ELISA (enzyme-linked immunosorbent assay) tests appear to be the best laboratory methods currently available.

Dealing with Food Allergies

Once a food allergy has been determined, the simplest and most effective method of dealing with it is through avoidance. Avoidance means not only avoiding the food in its most identifiable state (such as eggs in an omelet), but also in its hidden state (eggs in bread). Closely related foods with similar components may also need to be eliminated (for example, rice and millet in patients with severe wheat allergy).

It is also important to eliminate food additives. Food additives are used to prevent spoiling or enhance flavor and include such substances as preservatives, artificial colors, artificial flavorings, and acidifiers. The FDA has approved the use of over 2,800 different food additives. Although the government has banned many synthetic food additives, it should not be assumed that all the additives currently used in our food supply are safe. A great number of synthetic food additives still in use are being linked to allergies and such diseases as depression, asthma, hyperactivity or learning disabilities in children, and migraine headaches.[13]

If a person has multiple food allergies, the so-called rotary diversified diet is the best method to follow. This diet is made up of a highly varied selection of foods which are eaten in a definite rotation, or order, to prevent the formation of new allergies and control preexisting ones. Tolerated foods are eaten at regularly spaced intervals of four to seven days. For example, if a person has wheat on Monday, they will have to wait until Friday to have anything with wheat in it again. This approach is based on the principle that infrequent consumption of tolerated foods is not likely to induce new allergies or increase any mild allergies. As tolerance for eliminated foods returns, they may be added back into the rotation schedule without reactivation of the allergy (this of course applies only to cyclic food allergies; fixed allergenic foods may never be eaten again).

In addition to rotating tolerated foods, food families must also be rotated. Foods, whether animal or vegetable, come in families. It is important to rotate food families because foods in one family can "cross-react" with allergy-inducing foods. Steady consumption of foods that are members of the same family can lead to allergies. Food families need not be as strictly rotated as individual foods. It is usually recommended to avoid eating members of the same food family two days in a row. Table 4.6 lists family classifications for edible plants and animals; a simplified four-day rotation diet plan is provided in Table 4.7.

Table 4.6   Edible Plant and Animal Kingdom Taxonomic List

Vegetables

Legumes	**Mustard**	**Parsley**	**Potato**
Beans	Broccoli	Anise	Chile
Cocoa beans	Brussels sprouts	Caraway	Eggplant
Lentils	Cabbage	Carrot	Peppers
Licorice	Cauliflower	Celery	Potatoes
Peanuts	Mustard	Coriander	Tobacco
Peas	Radish	Cuzmin	Tomato
Soybeans	Turnip	Parsley	
Tamarinds	Watercress		
Grass	**Lily**	**Laurel**	**Sunflower**
Barley	Asparagus	Avocado	Artichoke
Corn	Chives	Camphor	Lettuce
Oat	Garlic	Cinnamon	Sunflower
Rice	Leeks		
Rye	Onions		
Wheat			
Beet	**Buckwheat**		
Beet	Buckwheat		
Chard	Rhubarb		
Spinach			

Fruits

Gourds	**Plums**	**Citrus**	**Cashew**
Cantaloupe	Almond	Grapefruit	Cashews
Cucumber	Apricot	Lemon	Mango
Honeydew	Cherry	Lime	Pistachio
Melons	Peach	Mandarin	
Pumpkin	Persimmon	Orange	
Squash	Plum	Tangerine	
Zucchini			
Nuts	**Beech**	**Banana**	**Palm**
Brazil nuts	Beechnuts	Arrowroot	Coconut
Pecans	Chestnuts	Banana	Date
Walnuts	Chinquapin nuts	Plantain	Date sugar

Table 4.6   *(continued)*

Grape	Pineapple	Rose	Birch
Grape	Pineapple	Blackberry	Filberts
Raisin		Loganberry	Hazelnuts
		Raspberry	
		Rose hips	
		Strawberry	

Apple	Blueberry	Pawpaws	
Apple	Blueberry	Papaya	
Pear	Cranberry	Pawpaw	
Quince	Huckleberry		

Animals

Mammals (Meat/Milk)	Birds (Meat/Egg)	Fish	
Cow	Chicken	Catfish	Salmon
Goat	Duck	Cod	Sardine
Pig	Goose	Flounder	Snapper
Rabbit	Hen	Halibut	Trout
Sheep	Turkey	Mackerel	Tuna

Crustaceans	Mollusks
Crab	Abalone
Crayfish	Clams
Lobster	Mussels
Prawn	Oysters
Shrimp	Scallops

*The names of food families are shown in this table in boldface.

Table 4.7   Four-Day Rotation Diet

Food Family	Food
Day 1	
Citrus	Lemon, orange, grapefruit, lime, tangerine, kumquat, citron
Banana	Banana, plantain, arrowroot (musa)
Palm	Coconut, date, date sugar

Table 4.7   (continued)

Food Family	Food
Day 1 (cont.)	
Parsley	Carrots, parsnips, celery, celery seed, celeriac, anise, dill, fennel, cumin, parsley, coriander, caraway
Spices	Black and white pepper, peppercorn, nutmeg, mace
Subucaya	Brazil nut
Bird	All fowl and game birds, including chicken, turkey, duck, goose, guinea, pigeon, quail, pheasant, eggs
Juices	Juices (preferably fresh) may be made and used from any fruits and vegetables listed above, in any combination desired, without adding sweeteners.
Day 2	
Grape	All varieties of grapes, raisin
Pineapple	Juice-pack, water-pack, or fresh
Rose	Strawberry, raspberry, blackberry, loganberry, rose hips
Gourd	Watermelon, cucumber, cantaloupe, pumpkin, squash, other melons, zucchini, pumpkin or squash seeds
Beet	Beet, spinach, chard
Legume	Peas, black-eyed peas, dry beans, green beans, carob, soybeans, lentils, licorice, peanuts, alfalfa
Cashew	Cashew, pistachio, mango
Birch	Filbert, hazelnut
Flaxseed	Flaxseed
Swine	All pork products
Mollusks	Abalone, snail, squid, clam, mussel, oyster, scallop
Crustaceans	Crab, crayfish, lobster, prawn, shrimp
Juices	Juices (preferably fresh) may be made and used without added sweeteners from any fruits, berries, or vegetables listed above, in any combination desired, including fresh alfalfa and some legumes.
Day 3	
Apple	Apple, pear, quince
Gooseberry	Currant, gooseberry
Buckwheat	Buckwheat, rhubarb

Table 4.7 *(continued)*

Food Family	Food
Day 3 (cont.)	
Aster	Lettuce, chicory, endive, escarole, globe artichoke, dandelion, sunflower seeds, tarragon
Potato	Potato, tomato, eggplant, peppers (red and green), chile pepper, paprika, cayenne, ground cherries
Lily (onion)	Onion, garlic, asparagus, chives, leeks
Spurge	Tapioca
Herb	Basil, savory, sage, oregano, horehound, catnip, spearmint, peppermint, thyme, marjoram, lemon balm
Walnut	English walnut, black walnut, pecan, hickory nut, butternut
Pedalium	Sesame
Beech	Chestnut
Saltwater fish	Herring, anchovy, cod, sea bass, sea trout, mackerel, tuna, swordfish, flounder, sole
Freshwater fish	Sturgeon, salmon, whitefish, bass, perch
Juices	Juices (preferably fresh) may be made and used without added sweeteners from any fruits and vegetables listed above, in any combination.
Day 4	
Plum	Plum, cherry, peach, apricot, nectarine, almond, wild cherry
Blueberry	Blueberry, huckleberry, cranberry, wintergreen
Pawpaws	Pawpaw, papaya, papain
Mustard	Mustard, turnip, radish, horseradish, watercress, cabbage, Chinese cabbage, broccoli, cauliflower, Brussels sprouts, kale, kohlrabi, rutabaga
Laurel	Avocado, cinnamon, bay leaf, sassafras, cassia buds or bark
Sweet potato or yam	
Grass	Wheat, corn, rice, oats, barley, rye, wild rice, cane, millet, sorghum, bamboo sprouts
Orchid	Vanilla
Protea	Macadamia nut

Table 4.7   *(continued)*

Food Family	Food
Day 4 (cont.)	
Conifer	Pine nut
Fungus	Mushrooms and yeast (brewer's yeast, etc.)
Bovid	Milk products—butter, cheese, yogurt, beef and milk products, oleomargarine, lamb
Juices	Juices (preferably fresh) may be made and used without added sweeteners from any fruits and vegetables listed above, in any combination desired.

Chapter Summary

Individuals suffering from stress or anxiety need to support the biochemistry of the body by following some important dietary guidelines. Specifically, they will gain the most benefit if they:

1. Eliminate or restrict the intake of caffeine.
2. Eliminate or restrict the intake of alcohol.
3. Eliminate refined carbohydrates from the diet.
4. Design a healthful diet.
5. Eat regular planned meals in a relaxed environment.
6. Control food allergies.

5

Exercise and Stress Reduction

The immediate effect of exercise is stress on the body; however, with a regular exercise program the body adapts. The body's response to this regular stress is that it becomes stronger, functions more efficiently, and has greater endurance. Exercise is a vital component of a comprehensive stress management program and overall good health.

Physical Benefits

The entire body benefits from regular exercise largely as a result of improved cardiovascular and respiratory function. Simply stated, exercise enhances the transport of oxygen and nutrients into cells. At the same time, exercise enhances the transport of carbon dioxide and waste products from the tissues of the body to the bloodstream and ultimately to eliminative organs.

Regular exercise is particularly important in reducing the risk of heart disease. It does this by lowering cholesterol levels, improving blood and oxygen supply to the heart, increasing the functional capacity of the heart, reducing blood pressure, reducing obesity, and exerting a favorable effect on blood clotting.[1]

Regular exercise increases stamina and energy levels. People who exercise regularly are much less likely to suffer from fatigue and depression.

Anti-Stress Benefits

Tension, depression, feelings of inadequacy, and worries diminish greatly with regular exercise. Exercise alone has been demonstrated to have a tremendous impact on improving mood and the ability to handle stressful situations.

In a study published in the *American Journal of Epidemiology* it was found that increased participation in exercise, sports, and physical activities is strongly associated with decreased symptoms of anxiety (restlessness, tension), depression (feelings that life is not worthwhile, low spirits), and malaise (rundown feeling, insomnia).[2]

Increased Endorphin Levels

Regular exercise has been shown to enhance powerful mood-elevating substances in the brain known as endorphins. These compounds exert similar effects to morphine. In fact, the name (*endo* = endogenous, or within the body; *-rphins* = morphines) was given because of the morphine-like effects. There is a clear association between exercise and endorphin elevation, and when endorphins go up, mood follows.[3]

Dennis Lobstein, Ph.D., a professor of exercise psychobiology at the University of New Mexico, compared the beta-endorphin levels and depression profiles of 10 joggers versus 10 sedentary men of the same age.[4] The sedentary men tested out more depressed, perceived greater stress in their lives, had more stress-circulating hormones and lower levels of beta-endorphins. As Dr. Lobstein stated, this "reaffirms that depression is very sensitive to exercise and helps firm up a biochemical link between physical activity and depression."[4]

Health Benefits of Regular Exercise

- Improved cardiovascular function as noted by a decreased heart rate, improved heart contraction, reduced blood pressure, and decreased blood cholesterol levels
- Enhanced immune function, especially natural killer cell activity
- Reduced secretions of adrenaline and noradrenaline in response to psychological stress
- Improved oxygen and nutrient utilization in all tissues
- Increased self-esteem, mood, and frame of mind
- Increased endurance and energy levels

How to Start an Exercise Program

First, make sure you are fit enough to start an exercise program. If you have been mostly inactive for a number of years or have a previously diagnosed illness, see your physician first.

If you are fit enough to begin, the next thing to do is find an activity that you will enjoy. The best exercises are the kind that get your heart moving. Aerobic activities such as walking briskly, jogging, bicycling, cross-country skiing, swimming, aerobic dance, and racquet sports are good examples. Brisk walking (5 miles an hour) for approximately 30 minutes at a time may be the very best form of exercise for weight loss. Walking can be done anywhere; it doesn't require any expensive equipment, just comfortable clothing and well-fitting shoes; and the risk for injury is extremely low. Exercise draws from all of the fat stores of the body, not just from local deposits of the body parts being used. While aerobic exercise generally enhances weight loss programs, weight training programs can also substantially alter body composition, by increasing lean body weight and decreasing body fat. Thus, weight training may be just as, or more, effective than aerobic exercise in maintaining or increasing lean body weight.

Intensity of Exercise

Exercise intensity is determined by measuring your heart rate (the number of times your heart beats per minute). This determination can be quickly done by placing the index and middle finger of one hand on the side of the neck just below the angle of the jaw or on the opposite wrist. Beginning with zero, count the number of heartbeats for 6 seconds. Simply add a zero to this number and you have your pulse. For example, if you counted 14 beats, your heart rate is 140. Is this a good number? It depends upon your "training zone."

A quick and easy way to determine your maximum training heart rate is to simply subtract your age from 185. For example, if you are 40 years old your maximum heart rate would be 145. To determine the bottom of the training zone, subtract 20. In the case of a 40-year-old, the number is 125. The training range for that person is a heartbeat between 125 and 145 beats per minute. For maximum health benefits you will want to stay in this range and never exceed it.

Duration and Frequency

A minimum of 15 to 20 minutes of exercising at your training heart rate at least three times a week is necessary to gain any significant cardiovascular benefits from exercise. It is better to exercise at the lower end of your training zone for longer periods of time than it is to exercise at a higher intensity for a shorter period of time. It is best if you can make exercise a part of your daily routine.

Make Exercise Fun

The key to getting the maximum benefit from exercise is to make it enjoyable. Choose an activity that you enjoy and have fun with. If you can find enjoyment in exercise, you are much more likely to do it. You won't get in good physical condition by exercising just once; it must be performed on a regular basis. So, make it fun.

Chapter Summary

Exercise is critical to good health and dealing with stress. Exercise not only strengthens the body, it also enhances mood and the ability to deal with stress. Exercise increases natural, mood-elevating substances in the brain known as endorphins. The key to gaining the benefits of exercise are to exercise on a regular basis and make it an enjoyable experience.

6

Nutritional and
Herbal Support

Nutritional and herbal support for the individual experiencing signs and symptoms of stress largely involves supporting the adrenal glands—two small glands which lie above each kidney. The adrenal glands control many body functions and play a critical role in resistance to stress. If an individual has experienced a great deal of stress or has taken corticosteroids for a long period of time, the adrenal glands will shrink and not perform properly, causing the experience of anxiety, depression, or chronic fatigue.

The Adrenal Glands

The adrenal glands are composed of two distinct parts, the inner part, known as the adrenal medulla, and the outer layer, known as the adrenal cortex.

The adrenal medulla secretes the hormones epinephrine (adrenaline) and norepinephrine (noradrenaline). In addition to playing a critical role in the so-called fight or flight response, these hormones also serve to maintain normal nervous control over many involuntary bodily functions such as heart rate, respiration, and digestion. The adrenal cortex secretes an entirely different group of hormones called corticosteroids. These hormones are all formed from cholesterol. Although all corticosteroids have similar chemical formulas, they differ in function. The three major types of corticosteroids are mineralocorticoids, glucocorticoids, and 17-ketosteroids (sex hormones).

The glucocorticoids, mainly cortisol, corticosterone and cortisone, exert a profound effect upon the metabolism of glucose. These hormones increase serum glucose. In addition, glucocorticoids reduce inflammation and the allergic response.

The mineralocorticoids, of which aldosterone is the most important, have a profound effect on minerals. Specifically, aldosterone increases the retention of sodium and the excretion of potassium by the body.

The 17-ketosteroids (sex hormones) are also secreted by the adrenals. The primary sex hormone produced by the adrenal is the androgen (male hormone), dehydroepiandrosterone (DHEA).

Stress and the Adrenals

An abnormal adrenal response, either deficient or excessive hormone release, significantly alters an individual's response to stress. Often the adrenals become "exhausted" as a result of constant demands placed upon them. An individual with adrenal exhaustion will usually suffer from chronic fatigue and may complain of feeling "stressed out" or anxious. They will typically have a reduced resistance to allergies and infection.

Atrophy (or shrinking) of the adrenal cortex is a common side effect of continual stress and cortisone administration. Because of the importance of the adrenal gland, optimal stress management is dependent on optimal adrenal function.

Supporting Adrenal Function

One of the best ways to support your adrenal glands is by learning how to effectively deal with stress through the regular use of relaxation techniques and exercise (see Chapters 3 and 5). In addition, the adrenal glands can be supported by eating a high-potassium diet along with taking nutritional supplements, adrenal extracts, and plant-based medicines like ginseng.

Foremost in the restoration or maintenance of proper adrenal function is to ensure adequate potassium levels within the body. This can best be done by consuming foods rich in potassium and avoiding foods high in sodium. Most Americans have a potassium-to-sodium (K:Na) ratio of less than 1:2. This means most people ingest twice as much sodium as potassium. Researchers recommend a dietary potassium-to-sodium ratio of greater than 5:1 to maintain health. This ratio is 10 times higher than the average intake. However, even this may not be optimal. A natural diet rich in fruits and vegetables can produce a K:Na ratio greater than 50:1, as most fruits and vegetables have a K:Na ratio of at least 100:1. For example, here are the average K:Na ratios for several common fresh fruits and vegetables:

carrots	75:1
potatoes	110:1
apples	90:1

bananas   440:1
oranges   260:1

To support the adrenals, the daily intake of potassium should be at least 3 to 5 grams per day. Table 6.1 lists some foods having a high content of potassium.

High-Potency Multiple Vitamin-Mineral Formulas

In an effort to increase their intake of essential nutrients, many Americans look to multiple vitamin and mineral supplements. In 1991 alone, over $400 million was spent on such products.

Tremendous scientific evidence supports the use of nutritional supplementation, but many medical experts have not overwhelmingly endorsed the concept. Some say diet alone can provide all the essential nutrition necessary, while many others will tout the health benefits of vitamins and minerals. The consumer is left in the middle trying to figure out which side is right.

First of all, to an extent, both sides are right. What it boils down to is what criteria of "optimum" nutrition is being used. If an expert believes optimum nutrition only means no obvious signs of nutrient deficiency, the answer to whether supplementation is necessary is going to be different from an expert who thinks of optimum nutrition as that which will allow a person to function at the highest level possible—with vitality, energy, and enthusiasm for living. What it comes down to then is a difference of philosophy.

Do you believe that health simply means not being sick? Or do you think health is much more than this? It is the goal of optimal health that drives people to take nutritional supplements.

Table 6.1   Potassium Content of Selected Foods

Milligrams (mg) per 100 grams edible portion (100 grams = 3.5 ounces)

Food	mg	Food	mg
Dulse	8,060	Cauliflower	295
Kelp	5,273	Watercress	282
Sunflower seeds	920	Asparagus	278
Wheat germ	827	Red cabbage	268
Almonds	773	Lettuce	264
Raisins	763	Cantaloupe	251
Parsley	727	Lentils, cooked	249
Brazil nuts	715	Tomato	244
Peanuts	674	Sweet potatoes	243
Dates	648	Papayas	234
Figs, dried	640	Eggplant	214
Avocados	604	Green peppers	213
Pecans	603	Beets	208
Yams	600	Peaches	202
Swiss chard	550	Summer squash	202
Soybeans, cooked	540	Oranges	200
Garlic	529	Raspberries	199
Spinach	470	Cherries	191
English walnuts	450	Strawberries	164
Millet	430	Grapefruit juice	162
Beans, cooked	416	Cucumbers	160
Mushrooms	414	Grapes	158
Potato with skin	407	Onions	157
Broccoli	382	Pineapple	146
Kale	378	Milk, whole	144
Bananas	370	Lemon juice	141
Meats	370	Pears	130
Winter squash	369	Eggs	129
Chicken	366	Apples	110
Carrots	341	Watermelon	100
Celery	341	Brown rice, cooked	70
Radishes	322		

Source: "Nutritive Value of American Foods in Common Units," *USDA Agriculture Handbook No. 456*

Who Takes Vitamins?

Taking vitamin and mineral supplements has become a way of life for many Americans. Data from the first and second United States Health and Nutrition Examination Survey (HANES I and II) conducted in the 1970s indicated that almost 35% of the U.S. population between 18 and 74 years of age were taking vitamin or mineral supplements regularly.[1] During the 1980s and early 1990s it is estimated that number has nearly doubled so that now over 60% of Americans take vitamin or mineral supplements.

Although somewhat outdated, the HANES data demonstrate some interesting facts about supplement users.[1] Perhaps the most interesting finding was that persons with the highest dietary nutrient intakes are the most likely to take a multiple vitamin and mineral supplement. This is extremely significant, as it says a great deal about how these individuals view optimum nutrition. They are not using nutritional supplements to replace a nutrient-poor diet. Instead, they are using supplements truly as they are intended, to supplement a good healthy diet.

Other interesting findings: college-educated individuals are much more likely to take a multiple supplement than those with less education; more women take supplements than men; supplement use is highest in the West and lowest in the South; individuals of normal weight or less are more likely to take supplements than heavier individuals; and individuals who exercise regularly are more likely to take a supplement than those who do not exercise regularly.

The Need for Nutritional Supplementation

Most Americans consume a diet inadequate in nutritional value yet not to a point where obvious nutrient deficiencies are apparent. The term "subclinical," or marginal, deficiency is often used to describe this situation. A subclinical deficiency indicates a deficiency of a particular vitamin or mineral that is not severe enough to produce a classic deficiency sign or symptom. Complicating the matter is that in many instances the only clue of a subclinical nutrient deficiency may be fatigue, lethargy, difficulty in concentrating, a lack of well-being, or some other vague symptom. Diagnosis of subclinical deficiencies is an extremely difficult process that involves detailed dietary or laboratory analysis.

Is there evidence to support the contention that subclinical vitamin and mineral deficiencies exist? Definitely yes. During recent years the U.S. government has sponsored a number of comprehensive studies (HANES I and II, Ten-State Nutrition Survey, USDA nationwide food consumption studies and others) to determine the nutritional status of the population. These studies have revealed that marginal nutrient deficiencies exist in a substantial portion of the U.S. population (approximately 50%) and that for some selected nutrients in certain age groups more than 80% of the group consumed less than the recommended dietary allowance (RDA).[2]

These studies indicate that the chances of consuming a diet meeting the RDA for all nutrients is extremely unlikely for most Americans. In other words, while it is theoretically possible that a healthy individual can get all the nutrition they need from foods, the fact is that most Americans do not even come close. Therefore, nutritional supplementation is essential.

Is the RDA Enough? Recommended dietary allowances for vitamins and minerals have been prepared by the Food and Nutrition Board of the National Research Council since 1941.[3] These guidelines were originally developed to reduce the rates of severe nutritional-deficiency diseases such as scurvy (deficiency of vitamin C), pellagra (deficiency of niacin) and beriberi (deficiency of vitamin B1). The RDAs were designed to serve as the basis for evaluating the adequacy of diets of groups of people, not individuals, who vary too widely in their nutritional requirements. As stated by the Food and Nutrition Board, "Individuals with special nutritional needs are not covered by the RDAs."

A tremendous amount of scientific research indicates that the optimal level for many nutrients, especially the so-called antioxidant nutrients like vitamins C and E, beta-carotene, and selenium, may be much higher than their current RDA. Another factor the RDAs do not adequately take into consideration are environmental and lifestyle factors which can destroy vitamins and bind minerals. For example, even the Food and Nutrition Board acknowledges that smokers require at least twice as much vitamin C compared to nonsmokers.[3] But what about other nutrients and smoking? And what about the effects of alcohol consumption, food additives, heavy metals (lead, mercury, etc.), carbon monoxide, and other chemicals associated with our modern society, which are known to interfere with nutrient function? Dealing with the varied hazards of modern living may be another reason why many people take supplements.

While the RDAs have done a good job at defining nutrient intake levels to prevent nutritional deficiencies, there is still much to be learned regarding the optimum intake of nutrients.

Multiple Vitamin-Mineral Formulas

The first thing to look for when selecting a multiple formula is to make sure that it provides the full range of vitamins and minerals. There are 13 different known vitamins, each with its own special role to play. The vitamins are classified into two groups: fat-soluble (A, D, E, and K) and water-soluble (the B vitamins and vitamin C). Vitamins function along with enzymes in chemical reactions necessary for human bodily function, including energy production. Together, vitamins and enzymes act as catalysts in speeding up the making or breaking of chemical bonds that join molecules together. Twenty-two different minerals are important in human nutrition. Minerals function along with vitamins as components of body enzymes and are also needed for proper composition of bone, blood, and the maintenance of normal cell function.

The following recommendations for the daily intake levels of vitamins and minerals are designed to provide an optimum intake range for maintaining health and supporting the adrenal glands. These recommended levels are most easily attained by taking a good multiple vitamin-mineral formula and then adding specific nutrients, like vitamin C and pantothenic acid, as needed.

Vitamin	*Daily Optimal Supplementation Range for Adults*
Vitamin A (retinol)	5,000–10,000 IU
Vitamin A (from beta-carotene)	10,000–75,000 IU
Vitamin D	100–400 IU
Vitamin E (d-alpha tocopherol)	400–1,200 IU
Vitamin K (phytonadione)	60–900 mcg
Vitamin C (ascorbic acid)	3,000–9,000 mg
Vitamin B1 (thiamin)	10–90 mg
Vitamin B2 (riboflavin)	10–90 mg
Niacin	10–90 mg
Niacinamide	10–30 mg
Vitamin B6 (pyridoxine)	25–100 mg
Biotin	100–300 mcg
Pantothenic acid	100–500 mg
Folic acid	400–1,000 mcg
Vitamin B12	400–1,000 mcg

Choline	150–500 mg
Inositol	150–500 mg

Minerals	*Daily Supplementation Range for Adults*
Boron	1–2 mg
Calcium	250–750 mg
Chromium	200–400 mcg
Copper	1–2 mg
Iodine	50–150 mcg
Iron	15–30 mg
Magnesium	500–750 mg
Manganese	10–15 mg
Molybdenum	10–25 mcg
Potassium	200–500 mg
Selenium	100–200 mcg
Silica	200–1,000 mcg
Vanadium	50–100 mcg
Zinc	15–30 mg

Key Nutrients

Several nutrients are especially important in supporting adrenal function: vitamin C, vitamin B6, zinc, magnesium, and pantothenic acid. All of these nutrients play a critical role in the health of the adrenal glands as well as the manufacture of adrenal hormones. Evidence indicates that during times of stress, the levels of these nutrients in the adrenals can plummet.

For example, it is well known that during times of chemical, emotional, psychological, or physiological stress, the urinary excretion of vitamin C is increased, signifying an increased need for vitamin C during these times.[4] Examples of chemical stressors include cigarette smoke, pollutants, and allergens. Extra vitamin C in the form of supplementation along with an increased intake of vitamin C-rich foods is often recommended to keep the immune system working properly during times of stress.

Equally important during high periods of stress or in individuals needing adrenal support is pantothenic acid (B vitamins). Pantothenic acid deficiency results in adrenal atrophy, which is characterized by fatigue, headache, sleep disturbances, nausea, and abdominal discomfort.[5] Pantothenic acid is found in whole grains, legumes, cauliflower, broccoli, salmon, liver, sweet potatoes, and tomatoes. In addition, it is a good idea to take at least an additional 100 milligrams of pantothenic acid daily. In patients suffering from chronic stress or a history of corticosteroid (prednisone) use, I recommend supplementing the diet with 500 milligrams of pantothenic acid daily.

The other key nutrients—vitamin B6, zinc, and magnesium—should also be taken at these levels.

Plant-Based Medicines

Numerous herbs support adrenal function. Most notable are the ginsengs. Both Chinese ginseng (*Panax ginseng*) and Siberian ginseng (*Eleutherococcus senticosus*) exert beneficial effects on adrenal function and enhance resistance to stress. These ginsengs are often referred to as general tonics or adaptogens.

The term general tonic implies that an herb will increase the overall tone of the whole body. The ginsengs are also often referred to as adrenal tonics because they can increase the tone and function of the adrenal glands. Panax and Siberian ginseng can be used to: restore vitality in debilitated and feeble individuals; increase feelings of energy; increase mental and physical performance; prevent the negative effects of stress and enhance the body's response to stress; offset some of the negative effects of cortisone; enhance liver function; and protect against radiation damage. All of these applications are backed up by good clinical research.[6-8]

The modern term *adaptogen* is a more descriptive term used to describe the general tonic effects of Siberian and Panax ginseng. An adaptogen is defined as a substance that: (1) must be innocuous and cause minimal disorders in the physiological functions of an organism; (2) must have a nonspecific action (it should increase resistance to adverse influences by a wide range of physical, chemical, and biochemical factors); and (3) usually has a normalizing action irrespective of the direction of the pathologic state. According to tradition and scientific evidence, both Siberian and Panax ginseng possess this kind of equilibrating, tonic, antistress action. Adaptogen describes its general effects quite well.

The ginsengs have been shown to enhance the ability to cope with various stressors, both physical and mental.[6-8] Presumably this anti-stress action is mediated by mechanisms that control the adrenal glands. Ginseng delays the onset and reduces the severity of the alarm phase response of the general adaptation syndrome.

People taking either of the ginsengs typically report an increased sense of well-being. Clinical studies have confirmed that both Siberian and Panax ginseng significantly reduce feelings of stress and anxiety.[6-8] For example, in one double-blind clinical study, nurses who had switched from day to night duty rated themselves for competence, mood, and general well-being, and were given a test for mental and physical performance, along with blood cell counts and blood chemistry evaluation.[9] The group who were given Panax ginseng demonstrated higher scores in competence, mood parameters, and mental and physical performance when compared with those receiving placebos. The nurses taking the ginseng felt more alert, yet more tranquil, and were able to perform better than the nurses not taking the ginseng.

In addition to these human studies, several animal studies have shown the ginsengs to exert significant anti-anxiety effects. In several of these studies, the stress-relieving effects were comparable to diazepam (Valium), however, while diazepam causes behavior changes, sedative effects, and impaired motor activity, ginseng produces none of these negative effects.[6,7,10]

Based on these clinical and animal studies, it appears that ginseng offers significant benefit to people suffering from stress and anxiety. Ginseng, particularly Panax ginseng, can also help restore adrenal function in individuals who have been under severe stress or who have taken corticosteroids like prednisone.

Another key indication for the need of adrenal support is chronic fatigue. Both Panax and Siberian ginseng have been shown to enhance energy levels. Some of the first studies of Panax and Siberian ginseng's energy-enhancing activities were performed during the late 1950s and early 1960s by Russian pharmacologist I.I. Brekhman.[6]

In one of Brekhman's experiments, Soviet soldiers given an extract of ginseng ran faster in a race than those given a placebo. In another, radio operators tested after administration of ginseng extract transmitted text significantly faster and with fewer mistakes than those given a placebo. These and similar results prompted other researchers to confirm the results in experimental models using mice.

In perhaps the best-known of these experiments, mice were subjected to swimming in cold water or running up an apparently endless rope to determine if ginseng could increase the time to exhaustion.[7] The results indicated that ginseng possessed significant anti-fatigue activity, as a clear dose-dependent increase in time to exhaustion was noted in mice who received ginseng. The higher the dose of ginseng, the longer the mice were able to swim.

The Right Ginseng

Panax ginseng is generally regarded as being more potent than Siberian ginseng. If you have been under a great deal of stress, or you are recovering from a long-standing illness, or you have taken corticosteroids like prednisone for a long period of time, the "best" ginseng for you is probably Panax ginseng. If you have been under mild to moderate stress and have less obvious impaired adrenal function, Siberian ginseng may be the best choice.

There are many types and grades of ginseng and ginseng extracts, depending on the source, age, and parts of the root used, and the methods of preparation. Unfortunately, for largely economic purposes, the majority of ginseng in the American marketplace is derived from the lowest grade root, diluted with excipients, blended with adulterants, or totally devoid of active ingredients.

High-quality ginseng extracts are available, however. For Panax ginseng, extracts that have been standardized for ginsenoside content and ratio (an Rg1 to Rb1 ratio of 1:2) to insure optimum pharmacological effect are preferred. The typical dose (taken one to three times daily) for individuals requiring adrenal support should contain a ginsenoside content of at least 15 milligrams. For example, the dosage for a 15% ginsenoside extract would be 100 milligrams, one to three times daily. Lower doses can be used as a general tonic.

Siberian ginseng is typically standardized for its eleutheroside E content (greater than 1%) because there is a good correlation between this constituent and the quality and activity of the extract. Typical dosage is 100 milligrams of this extract three times daily.

As each individual's response to ginseng is unique, it is best to begin at lower doses and increase gradually. The Russian approach for long-term administration is to use ginseng cyclically for a period of 15 to 20 days followed by a two-week interval without any ginseng.

Too much ginseng may cause a number of side effects including anxiety, irritability, nervousness, insomnia, hypertension, breast pain, and menstrual changes. If any of these side effects appear, the dosage should be reduced or the product discontinued.

Adrenal Extracts

If additional adrenal support is required, oral adrenal extracts made from beef can be used to nourish and support adrenal function. Adrenal extracts have been used in medicine since 1931.[11] Adrenal extracts may be made from the whole adrenal or from the adrenal cortex only. Whole adrenal extracts (usually in combination with essential nutrients for the adrenal gland) are used most often in cases of low adrenal function present as chronic fatigue, inability to cope with stress, and reduced resistance. Because extracts made from the adrenal cortex contain small amounts of corticosteroids, they are typically used as a "natural" cortisone in severe cases of allergy and inflammation (asthma, eczema, psoriasis, rheumatoid arthritis, etc.).

I recommend using the whole adrenal extract. The dosage of adrenal extract will depend upon the quality and potency of the product. The best measure of an effective dose for either preparation may be the level of stimulation experienced. If a high-quality preparation is used, at higher dosages (for example, twice the label recommendation) a general stimulatory effect will be noticed and may include irritability, restlessness, and insomnia. I suggest starting at one-third the recommended dosage on the label and slowly increasing the amount every two days until you notice the stimulatory effect. Once you notice this effect, reduce the dosage to just below that level that produces excess stimulation. As your adrenal glands rebuild, reduce the amount you take until you do not require the additional support.

Chapter Summary

The adrenal glands control many bodily functions and play a critical role in the resistance to stress. If an individual has experienced a great deal of stress or has taken corticosteroids for a long period of time, the adrenal glands will shrink and not perform properly, causing chronic fatigue, reduced resistance, and allergies. The adrenal glands can be supported by learning how to deal effectively with stress: through the regular use of relaxation techniques and exercise, by eating a high-potassium diet, and taking nutritional supplements, adrenal extracts, and ginseng.

Anxiety

7

Understanding Anxiety

Anxiety is defined as "an unpleasant emotional state ranging from mild unease to intense fear." Anxiety differs from fear in that fear is a rational response to a real danger, and anxiety usually lacks a clear or realistic cause. Though some anxiety is normal and in fact healthy, higher levels of anxiety are uncomfortable and can lead to significant problems.

Anxiety is often accompanied by a variety of symptoms. The most common symptoms are heart palpitations (awareness of a more forceful or faster heart beat), throbbing or stabbing pains in the chest, a feeling of tightness and inability to take in enough air, and a tendency to sigh or hyperventilate. Tension in the muscles of the back and neck often leads to headaches, back pains, and muscle spasms. Other symptoms can include excessive sweating, dryness of the mouth, dizziness, digestive disturbances, and the constant need to urinate or defecate.

Anxious individuals usually have a constant feeling that something bad is going to happen. They may fear that they have a chronic or dangerous illness, a belief that is reinforced by the symptoms of anxiety. Inability to relax may lead to difficulty in getting to sleep and constant waking throughout the night.

Panic Attacks

Severe anxiety will often produce what are known as "panic attacks"—intense feelings of fear. Panic attacks may occur independent of anxiety, but are most often associated with generalized anxiety or agoraphobia, an intense fear of being alone or being in public places. As a result, most people with agoraphobia become housebound.

How common are panic attacks? Very. Results from a recent survey published in the *American Journal of Psychiatry* indicate that about 15% of the United States population experience a panic attack in their lifetimes, and 3% reported a panic attack in the preceding month.[1] These results and others indicate that panic attacks are much more common than previously thought. It is now estimated that among adults aged 25 to 54 years, the prevalence of panic attacks is roughly between 1.5% and 3% of the population.

Causes of Anxiety and Panic Attacks

Clinical anxiety, including panic attacks, can be produced by caffeine, certain other drugs, and the infusion of lactate into the blood. Knowing that these compounds can produce anxiety and panic attacks can be put to good use in understanding the underlying biochemical features of anxiety.

Perhaps the most significant biochemical disturbance noted in patients with anxiety and panic attacks is an elevated blood lactate level and an increased lactate-to-pyruvate ratio. Lactate (the soluble form of lactic acid) is the final pathway in the breakdown of blood sugar (glucose) when there is a lack of oxygen.

To illustrate how lactic acid is produced, let's look at the classic example of the exercising muscle. Muscles prefer to use fat as the energy source, but when you exercise vigorously, there isn't enough oxygen so the muscle must burn glucose. Without oxygen, lactic acid builds up within the muscle—this is what causes muscle fatigue and soreness after exercise. Let's take a look at this process.

The first few steps of normal glucose breakdown can be done without oxygen, until pyruvate is produced (Figure 7.1).

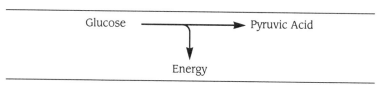

Figure 7.1

The next steps require oxygen and end up in the complete breakdown of pyruvic acid to carbon dioxide and water (Figure 7.2).

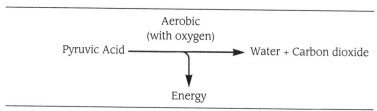

Figure 7.2

But what happens if there is not enough oxygen? The exercising muscle will need energy, so the muscle cell converts as much glucose to pyruvic acid as possible. This process is referred to as *anaerobic metabolism*. The pyruvic acid is converted to a temporary waste product—lactic acid (Figure 7.3).

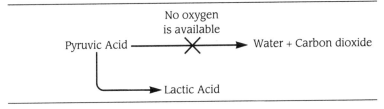

Figure 7.3

With good circulation, the lactic acid is removed from the muscle and transported to the liver where it can either be turned back into pyruvic acid or even back to glucose if needed (Figure 7.4).

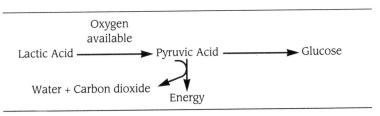

Figure 7.4

How does all this biochemistry relate to anxiety? Individuals with anxiety have elevated blood levels of lactate and higher levels of lactate to pyruvate compared to normal controls. Furthermore, in patients with panic attacks (a severe anxiety reaction), who are injected with lactate, more severe panic attacks are produced. In normal individuals nothing happens. It appears that individuals with anxiety are sensitive to lactate. In other words, lactate may be causing anxiety.

Reducing the level of lactate is a critical goal in the treatment of anxiety and panic attacks. Achieving this goal is discussed in Chapter 8, "The Natural Approach to Anxiety and Panic Attacks."

The Standard Medical Approach

When most people go to a medical doctor or psychiatrist for relief of symptoms of anxiety they are usually given either a benzodiazepine (tranquilizer) or an antidepressant like Prozac. Very rarely are underlying factors or non-drug measures discussed.

The influence that the pharmaceutical industry has on medical thought is perhaps most evident in the treatment of psychological disorders. A recent editorial in the medical journal *Biological Psychiatry* summarizes this influence and what comes with it:

"The overall influence of the industry is to emphasize drug treatment at the expense of other modalities: psychotherapy, social approaches, nutritional, herbal, and natural remedies, rehabilitation, general hygienic measures, non-patentable drugs, or other alternative approaches. It focuses attention on disorders that are treatable by drugs, and may promote overdiagnosis. It reinforces the practice of dealing with disease by treatment of symptoms, and diverts interest from prevention."[2]

It is much easier from the physician's perspective to write out a prescription than to try to figure out what psychological or physiological factors may be causing the anxiety.

While tranquilizers and antidepressants are often effective in reducing the anxiety, they do not address the underlying cause. Tranquilizers are also highly addictive. Before drug treatment is used, I believe the anxious person should try the non-drug treatments detailed throughout this book, as well as psychological counseling.

The current drug treatments for anxiety and panic disorders are far from ideal. To illustrate the potential risk of relying on the drug approach, let's examine the benzodiazepines and Prozac more closely.

Benzodiazepines

The benzodiazepine drugs such as triazolam (Halcion), diazepam (Valium), and chlordiazepoxide (Librium) have become the the primary drugs prescribed for anxiety as well as insomnia. Other drugs in this category include: loazepam (Ativan), prazepam (Centrax), flurazepam (Dalmane), clonazepam (Klonopin), halazepam (Paxipam), tamazepam (Restoril), oxazepam (Serax), chloazepate (Tranxene), and alprazolam (Xanax).

The benzodiazepines induce sleep by enhancing the action of the nerve transmitter gamma-aminobutyric acid (GABA), which in turn blocks the arousal of brain centers. Benzodiazepines are not designed for long-term use, as they are addictive, associated with numerous side effects, and cause abnormal sleep patterns (discussed in more detail in Chapter 10).

The benzodiazepines can produce many side effects. Because the drugs can produce dizziness, drowsiness, and impaired coordination, it is important not to drive or engage in any potentially dangerous activities while on these drugs. Alcohol should never be consumed with benzodiazepines.

Benzodiazepines will often produce a morning "hangover" feeling. Other possible side effects include allergic reactions, headache, blurred vision, nausea, indigestion, diarrhea or constipation, and lethargy.

The most serious side effects of the benzodiazepines relate to their effects on memory and behavior. Because the drugs act on brain chemistry, significant changes in brain function and behavior can occur. This can manifest as severe memory impairment and amnesia of events while on the drug, nervousness, confusion, hallucinations, bizarre behavior, and extreme irritability and aggressiveness. Benzodiazepines have also been shown to increase feelings of depression, including suicidal thinking.

Benzodiazepines, especially Halcion, have been receiving a great deal of negative attention in the media the past few years. More people are "waking up" to the fact that these drugs can be quite dangerous if used for other than occasional use. If you have taken a benzodiazepine for more than four weeks, do not stop taking the drug suddenly. Work with your physician and taper off the drug gradually to avoid potentially dangerous withdrawal symptoms. Symptoms of withdrawal can include: anxiety, irritability, sensations of panic, insomnia, nausea, headache, impaired concentration, memory loss, depression, extreme sensitivity to the environment, seizures, hallucinations, and paranoia.

Prozac

The drug Prozac, the most commonly prescribed drug for depression, has been a topic of considerable interest in the national media of late. While some promote Prozac as a "wonder drug" others are quite concerned about the bizarre behavior the drug may induce.

Prozac and other antidepressants fit nicely into the dominant theoretical model of depression—the "biogenic amine" hypothesis. This model supposes that biochemical factors in the brain are causing depression rather than psychological factors. According to the biogenic amine hypothesis, depression is due to a biochemical derangement characterized by imbalances of amino acids which form neurotransmitters (compounds that transmit information to and from nerve cells).

Perhaps the main reason this model is so popular is that it is a good fit for drug therapy. The antidepressant drugs, as well as the use of amino acids like tryptophan and tyrosine, are designed to correct or lessen suspected imbalances in the biogenic amines (serotonin, melatonin, dopamine, epinephrine and norepinephrine). These compounds are also known as monoamines. The amino acid tryptophan serves as the precursor to serotonin and melatonin, while phenylalanine and tyrosine are precursors to dopamine, epinephrine and norepinephrine. Different antidepressant drugs act by increasing different monoamines in the brain.

Major Categories of Antidepressant Drugs
Bicyclic
    fluoxetine (Prozac)
Tricyclic
    amitryptaline (Elavil, Endep)
    desipramine (Norpramin, Pertofrane)
    doxepin (Adapin, Sinequan)
    imipramine (Imavate, Presamine, Trofinil)
    nortryptaline (Aventyl, Pamelor)
    protryptaline (Vivactil)
Monoamine oxidase inhibitors
    phenelzine (Nardil)
    tranylcypromine (Parnate)

While Prozac and other antidepressants may be successful in alleviating depression in many cases, they are also associated with many side effects, including increased nervousness, anxiety, insomnia, allergic reactions, and nausea. In addition, it is well accepted that Prozac causes a condition called akathisia in some patients. Akathisia is a drug-induced state of agitation, and in some people, it may induce truly violent and destructive outbursts.

The violent reactions experienced by some patients taking Prozac have been so common and publicized that several citizens groups have formed to create awareness of these dangers. Adverse reactions to the FDA-approved drug Prozac are alarmingly high.

The Citizen's Commission on Human Rights, through the Freedom of Information Act, received the adverse drug reaction reports on all of the major antidepressant drugs from 1985 to June 1992. During that time, Prozac received 23,067 claims of adverse drug reactions compared to Elavil, a commonly used standby antidepressant, which received only 2,032. Suicide attempts in the Elavil group were 10, compared to 1,436 attempts with Prozac, and death rates in the Prozac group were 1,313 compared to 159 for Elavil. Of course, because Prozac is more commonly prescribed, this could explain the increase, but serious, violent behavior associated with Prozac has even entered the courtroom in several cases.

Because of the negative publicity, the FDA convened a special committee to examine the growing concern about Prozac. This committee included 10 psychiatrists, but they appear to have been significantly biased in favor of the drug.

In the lengthy and insightful report titled "Prozac, Eli Lilly and the FDA" that appeared in the *Townsend Letter for Doctors* (February, 1993), Gary Null points out substantial evidence of committee bias.[3] For example, when Dr. Martin Teicher, a Harvard researcher, began to present substantial evidence of the link between Prozac and violent, suicidal thoughts at the FDA hearing, the panel refused to allow him to present his slides because they were not interested in his findings. Instead, the panel allowed three slide presentations in defense of Prozac.

The panel was not interested in some of the other points brought up by Dr. Teicher after he sat through the Eli Lilly-sponsored presentations. For example, in the presentation given by one psychiatrist sponsored by Eli Lilly, it was noted that the common risk factors associated with suicide are anxiety, insomnia, panic attacks, and poor concentration. Dr. Teicher pointed out that Eli Lilly's prescribing information for Prozac lists anxiety and insomnia as one of the most common side effects. During the drug's clinical trials, 9% of trial subjects receiving Prozac experienced anxiety and 13.8% experienced insomnia; these side effects were not noted in subjects taking the placebo. If anxiety and insomnia are risk factors for suicide and Prozac causes these side effects, there may be a link between Prozac and suicide. The FDA panel simply ignored Dr. Teicher when he pointed out the contradiction.

According to several experts in this matter, the FDA panel received enough evidence linking Prozac and violence to take action against the drug, but for some reason the panel chose not to.[4] Conflict of interest? Eight of the 10 panelists were psychiatrists, a profession that profits from Prozac. Other potential evidence of skewed science is that 9 of the 10 members had financial conflicts of interest. For example, one psychiatrist at the time he sat on the panel had already received $20,000 in grants from Sandoz, the manufacturer of Pamelor, the second most widely prescribed antidepressant.

Another psychiatrist who received $170,000 worth of grants from makers of antidepressants also gave positive reviews of two other antidepressant drugs in the 1980s—zimelidine and nomifensine. Within two years of his review, both drugs were pulled off the market due to serious side effects.

Another panel member had conflicts totaling half a million dollars from four manufacturers of antidepressants. Remarkably, this person also had $200,000 worth of grants "pending" from Eli Lilly, Prozac's maker, when the hearing took place. Upon review of the potential conflict of interest, the Citizen's Commission on Human Rights discovered that his conflict of interest waiver did not include several relevant items. This omission is serious as it violates federal laws.

The conflicts not disclosed in the waiver included the following: two pending grants worth $250,000 from antidepressant drug makers and an engagement to speak at a series of seminars funded by Eli Lilly. The psychiatrist failed to mention these conflicts; in fact in his waiver he stated that he had no current commitments to speak.

These omissions may have slipped his mind. But even without them, he certainly should have not been on the panel. After all, here was a situation where a psychiatrist had received over $4 million worth of research grants from antidepressant manufacturers in an eight-year period prior to being chosen to be on the FDA panel to discuss taking these very same drugs off the market. The potential conflict of interest is obvious.

Before Taking Prozac   It is important to realize there are other models and natural treatment options, as discussed in Chapters 8 and 10. Be sure that you really are depressed. Although nearly one of every four individuals experience some degree of clinical depression or mood disorder in their lifetime, effective relief is not dependent upon drug therapy. In fact, drug therapy for depression is only slightly better than a placebo. Most people are better off trying to work out their depression without drugs.

Clinical Depression

The official definition of "clinical" depression, as defined by the American Psychiatric Association in its *Diagnostic and Statistical Manual of Mental Disorders* (DSM-III) is based upon the following eight primary criteria:

1. Poor appetite with weight loss, or increased appetite with weight gain
2. Insomnia or hypersomnia
3. Physical hyperactivity or inactivity
4. Loss of interest or pleasure in usual activities, or decrease in sexual drive
5. Loss of energy and feelings of fatigue
6. Feelings of worthlessness, self-reproach, or inappropriate guilt
7. Diminished ability to think or concentrate
8. Recurrent thoughts of death or suicide

The presence of five of these eight symptoms definitely indicates depression; the individual with four is probably depressed. According to the DSM-III, the depressed state must be present for at least one month to be called depression. In many cases, depression is an appropriate response to a life event, and specific medical treatment is not needed.

Test Your Depression

If you have some symptoms of depression, you may want to take the test in Figure 7.5 developed by the Center for Epidemiological Studies of the National Institute of Mental Health. Circle the answer that best describes how you have felt over the past week.

During the past week:

1. I was bothered by things that usually don't bother me.
   - 0 *Rarely or none of the time (less than 1 day)*
   - 1 *Some or little of the time (1–2 days)*
   - 2 *Occasionally or a moderate amount of the time (3–4 days)*
   - 3 *Most or all of the time (5–7 days)*

2. I did not feel like eating; my appetite was poor.
   - 0 *Rarely or none of the time (less than 1 day)*
   - 1 *Some or little of the time (1–2 days)*
   - 2 *Occasionally or a moderate amount of the time (3–4 days)*
   - 3 *Most or all of the time (5–7 days)*

3. I felt that I could not shake off the blues even with help from my family and friends.
   - 0 *Rarely or none of the time (less than 1 day)*
   - 1 *Some or little of the time (1–2 days)*
   - 2 *Occasionally or a moderate amount of the time (3–4 days)*
   - 3 *Most or all of the time (5–7 days)*

4. I felt that I was not as good as other people.
   - 0 *Rarely or none of the time (less than 1 day)*
   - 1 *Some or little of the time (1–2 days)*
   - 2 *Occasionally or a moderate amount of the time (3–4 days)*
   - 3 *Most or all of the time (5–7 days)*

Figure 7.5 Test your depression

5. I had trouble keeping my mind on what I was doing.
   0   *Rarely or none of the time (less than 1 day)*
   1   *Some or little of the time (1–2 days)*
   2   *Occasionally or a moderate amount of the time (3–4 days)*
   3   *Most or all of the time (5–7 days)*

6. I felt depressed.
   0   *Rarely or none of the time (less than 1 day)*
   1   *Some or little of the time (1–2 days)*
   2   *Occasionally or a moderate amount of the time (3–4 days)*
   3   *Most or all of the time (5–7 days)*

7. I felt that everything I did was an effort.
   0   *Rarely or none of the time (less than 1 day)*
   1   *Some or little of the time (1–2 days)*
   2   *Occasionally or a moderate amount of the time (3–4 days)*
   3   *Most or all of the time (5–7 days)*

8. I felt hopeless about the future.
   0   *Rarely or none of the time (less than 1 day)*
   1   *Some or little of the time (1–2 days)*
   2   *Occasionally or a moderate amount of the time (3–4 days)*
   3   *Most or all of the time (5–7 days)*

9. I thought my life had been a failure.
   0   *Rarely or none of the time (less than 1 day)*
   1   *Some or little of the time (1–2 days)*
   2   *Occasionally or a moderate amount of the time (3–4 days)*
   3   *Most or all of the time (5–7 days)*

10. I felt fearful.
    0   *Rarely or none of the time (less than 1 day)*
    1   *Some or little of the time (1–2 days)*
    2   *Occasionally or a moderate amount of the time (3–4 days)*
    3   *Most or all of the time (5–7 days)*

11. My sleep was restless.
    0   *Rarely or none of the time (less than 1 day)*
    1   *Some or little of the time (1–2 days)*
    2   *Occasionally or a moderate amount of the time (3–4 days)*
    3   *Most or all of the time (5–7 days)*

12. I was unhappy.
    0   *Rarely or none of the time (less than 1 day)*
    1   *Some or little of the time (1–2 days)*
    2   *Occasionally or a moderate amount of the time (3–4 days)*
    3   *Most or all of the time (5–7 days)*

Figure 7.5 (continued)

13. I talked less than usual.
    - 0 *Rarely or none of the time (less than 1 day)*
    - 1 *Some or little of the time (1–2 days)*
    - 2 *Occasionally or a moderate amount of the time (3–4 days)*
    - 3 *Most or all of the time (5–7 days)*

14. I felt lonely.
    - 0 *Rarely or none of the time (less than 1 day)*
    - 1 *Some or little of the time (1–2 days)*
    - 2 *Occasionally or a moderate amount of the time (3–4 days)*
    - 3 *Most or all of the time (5–7 days)*

15. People were unfriendly.
    - 0 *Rarely or none of the time (less than 1 day)*
    - 1 *Some or little of the time (1–2 days)*
    - 2 *Occasionally or a moderate amount of the time (3–4 days)*
    - 3 *Most or all of the time (5–7 days)*

16. I did not enjoy life.
    - 0 *Rarely or none of the time (less than 1 day)*
    - 1 *Some or little of the time (1–2 days)*
    - 2 *Occasionally or a moderate amount of the time (3–4 days)*
    - 3 *Most or all of the time (5–7 days)*

17. I had crying spells.
    - 0 *Rarely or none of the time (less than 1 day)*
    - 1 *Some or little of the time (1–2 days)*
    - 2 *Occasionally or a moderate amount of the time (3–4 days)*
    - 3 *Most or all of the time (5–7 days)*

18. I felt sad.
    - 0 *Rarely or none of the time (less than 1 day)*
    - 1 *Some or little of the time (1–2 days)*
    - 2 *Occasionally or a moderate amount of the time (3–4 days)*
    - 3 *Most or all of the time (5–7 days)*

19. I felt that people disliked me.
    - 0 *Rarely or none of the time (less than 1 day)*
    - 1 *Some or little of the time (1–2 days)*
    - 2 *Occasionally or a moderate amount of the time (3–4 days)*
    - 3 *Most or all of the time (5–7 days)*

20. I could not get "going."
    - 0 *Rarely or none of the time (less than 1 day)*
    - 1 *Some or little of the time (1–2 days)*
    - 2 *Occasionally or a moderate amount of the time (3–4 days)*
    - 3 *Most or all of the time (5–7 days)*

Figure 7.5 (continued)

To Score Your Test

Add up the numbers you circled. If you scored from 0 to 9, it is extremely unlikely that you suffer from depression. A score of 10 to 15 puts you in the mildly depressed range, and 16 to 24 in the moderately depressed range. If you scored over 24, you probably suffer from clinical depression. However, unless you are considering suicide, I encourage you to follow the recommendations in Chapter 9. If you have seriously thought about suicide, I urge you to see a mental health specialist immediately.

Chapter Summary

Anxiety is defined as "an unpleasant emotional state ranging from mild unease to intense fear." Anxiety is often accompanied by a variety of physical symptoms. The most common symptoms are heart palpitations, throbbing or stabbing pains in the chest, a feeling of tightness and inability to take in enough air, and a tendency to sigh or hyperventilate.

Panic attacks are characterized by feelings of intense fear and are most often associated with anxiety or agoraphobia. Panic attacks and anxiety are characterized by an increase in the lactate-to-pyruvate ratio.

The standard medical approach focuses on drug treatment rather than addressing underlying factors and/or employing non-drug therapies. Benzodiazepines and antidepressant drugs are the most commonly used drugs in anxiety and panic disorders, but both carry with them clear risks and disadvantages.

8

The Natural Approach
to Anxiety

The natural approach to treating anxiety builds upon the treatments given for stress in Section I. Anxiety is often a symptom of severe stress. If you suffer from mild anxiety, follow the recommendations for calming the mind and body, and implementing a good diet, exercise, nutritional supplementation, and Panax ginseng. For moderate to severe anxiety, instead of Panax ginseng, try one of the natural anti-anxiety agents discussed in Chapter 9. In addition, follow the guidelines and recommendations presented in this chapter.

Lactate Levels and Anxiety

It was pointed out in the last chapter that increased lactic acid levels may be an underlying factor in panic attacks and anxiety. Our goal is to prevent the conversion of pyruvic acid to lactic acid and to aid the conversion of lactic acid back to pyruvate. Nutrition appears to play a key role in this goal. According to Melvyn Werbach, M.D., author of *Nutritional Influences on Mental Illness* (Third Line Press, 1991), at least six nutritional factors may be responsible for elevated lactate or lactate-to-pyruvate levels:[1]

1. Alcohol
2. Caffeine
3. Sugar
4. Deficiency of the B vitamins, niacin, pyridoxine, and thiamin
5. Deficiency of calcium or magnesium
6. Food allergies

By avoiding alcohol, caffeine, sugar, and food allergies a person with anxiety can go a long way in relieving his or her symptoms.[1] Simply not drinking coffee can result in complete elimination of symptoms. This recommendation may seem too simple to be true, but substantial clinical evidence indicates that in many cases it is all that is necessary. For example, in one study of four men and two women with generalized anxiety or panic disorder who were consuming the amount of caffeine in 1.5 to 3.5 cups of coffee per day, avoiding caffeine for one week brought about significant relief.[2] The degree of improvement was so noticeable that all patients volunteered to continue to abstain from coffee. Previously, these patients had been only minimally helped by drug therapy. Follow-up exams 6 to 18 months afterward indicated that five out of the six patients were completely without symptoms, and the sixth patient became asymptomatic with a very low dose of benzodiazepine.

By following the dietary guidelines given in Chapter 4 as well as the recommendations for nutritional supplementation given in Chapter 6, you will be providing your body with the kind of nutritional support necessary to counteract the biochemical derangements found in patients with anxiety and panic attacks.

Flaxseed Oil and Agoraphobia

The human body cannot function properly without two polyunsaturated fats—linoleic and alpha-linolenic acid. These fatty acids are referred to as essential fatty acids because they truly are essential to normal cell structure and body function. Agoraphobia may sometimes result from a deficiency of alpha-linolenic acid.

Both essential fatty acids function as components of nerve cells, cell membranes, and hormone-like substances known as prostaglandins. Although both linoleic acid and alpha-linolenic acid are 18-carbon-length fatty acids, alpha-linolenic acid has three unsaturated bonds while linoleic acid has only two. The location of the first unsaturated bond is different as well. Alpha-linolenic acid's first unsaturated bond occurs at the third carbon, hence it is known as an omega-3 oil. Linoleic acid's first double bond is at the sixth carbon, hence it is an omega-6 oil.

There is growing evidence that most Americans suffer from a relative deficiency of omega-3 oils. It is believed that the optimum ratio of omega-6 to omega-3 in our body tissues is somewhere around 4:1. However, analysis of tissue samples in many Americans has shown a common ratio of approximately 20:1.

Largely because linoleic acid and alpha-linolenic acid form entirely different prostaglandins, researchers and physicians are finding that by manipulating the type of dietary oils they can dramatically alter body function and, in some cases, treat disease. The omega-3 oils are showing the greatest promise in this regard.

In one study, three out of four patients with a history of agoraphobia for 10 or more years improved within two to three months after taking flaxseed oil at a dosage of 2 to 6 tablespoons daily (in divided doses depending upon response).[3] All patients had signs of essential fatty acid deficiency such as dry skin, dandruff, brittle fingernails that grow slowly, and nerve disorders.

High-Quality Flaxseed Oil   Not all flaxseed oil is created equal. Significant variation occurs in quality and purity due to differences in how the oil is expressed. Most flaxseed oils are produced by mechanically pressing out the oil through an expeller. During this process, a tremendous amount of pressure and heat can be generated. The higher the heat, the better the yield of oil. Temperatures generally reach 200 degrees Fahrenheit. Interestingly, flax oil processed in this manner can still be referred to as cold-pressed because no external source of heat was added.

Although high temperatures will provide a greater quantity of oil, they produce a lower quality oil. Many manufacturers will sacrifice quality for quantity. However, consumers must be aware that because flax oil is a highly polyunsaturated oil, it is extremely susceptible to damage by heat, light, and oxygen. Once damaged, the oil is a rich source of toxic molecules known as lipid peroxides. These molecules can actually do the body harm and should not be ingested. Lipid peroxides are associated with an extremely bitter taste and rancidity. One of the best ways to measure the quality of a flax oil is by taste. The degree of bitterness is a close approximation of the level of lipid peroxides.

A high-quality flaxseed oil will have a delicious, nutty flavor making it easy to incorporate into your daily diet as a salad dressing or flavoring. My wife and I pour 1 or 2 tablespoons over brown rice, cereal, or on our bread every day. My wife wouldn't do this unless it was health-promoting and good-tasting. (We use the Barlean's brand because we believe it is the best-tasting.)

Your best source of high-quality flaxseed oil will be health food stores. Most will offer several manufacturers to choose from. In general, most health food store brands are produced by special expeller extractions at temperatures below 96 degrees Fahrenheit, taking special care to protect the delicate oil from the damaging effects of heat, light, and oxygen.

Here are some general guidelines to follow in selecting a good flaxseed oil product:

1. Make sure the oil is derived from 100% third-party certified organic flaxseed. Oil expressed from non-organic seed may contain pesticides and herbicides.
2. Do not take the oil in capsule form. Your only assurance of quality is taste. Buy the oil in liquid form in opaque plastic bottles.
3. Make sure the oil is as fresh as possible and not past the expiration date.
4. Make sure it is clearly indicated that the oil is expeller-pressed.
5. To gain more benefit, use flaxseed oil high in lignan.

Another Model of Anxiety and Depression

In the previous chapter, the biogenic amine model of depression and anxiety was presented. This is the dominant model because it fits nicely with our society's typical drug approach to treating everything, but another model based on a social and psychological perspective does exist. The model was largely developed by Martin Seligman, Ph.D. In my opinion, what Einstein was to physics, Dr. Seligman is to social psychology. If you are interested in learning more about Dr. Seligman's work, I encourage you to read his book *Learned Optimism* published by Alfred A. Knopf (New York, 1991).

Dr. Seligman developed an animal model of depression known as the "learned helplessness model of depression." Basically, the animals were trained to be helpless; they had no control over their environment. Nothing they did would bring them relief from negative stimuli. As a result, the animals would simply give up. They would first become quite anxious then severely withdrawn and depressed.

Seligman followed up these animal experiments with human studies. Sure enough, after years of research Seligman and others were able to demonstrate that human anxiety and depression were symptoms of "learned helplessness." When animals learn to be helpless, biochemical changes occur in the brain. These biochemical changes can be reversed with the use of antidepressant drugs; in fact, the learned helplessness model is the premier model that drug companies use initially to test antidepressant drugs. Biochemical changes can also be reversed by teaching the animal how to regain control over its environment or situation. As the animal regains control over some aspects of their lives, its "depression" is lifted.

Human studies have shown the same results. While most physicians will quickly reach for the drug to alter brain chemistry, helping patients gain greater control over their lives will actually produce even greater biochemical changes.

Dr. Seligman used the phrase "learned optimism" when he and other researchers found a direct correlation between an individual's level of optimism and the likelihood of developing anxiety or clinical depression.[4,5] The patients were followed for a total of 35 years. While optimists rarely got anxious or depressed, pessimists were extremely likely to battle anxiety or depression.

Test Your Optimism

Dr. Seligman has developed a simple test to determine your level of optimism (Figure 7.6). Take as much time as you need to answer each of the questions. There are no right or wrong answers. It is important that you take the test before you read the interpretation. Read the description of each situation and vividly imagine it happening to you. Choose the response that most applies to you by circling either A or B. Ignore the letter and number codes for now, they will be explained later.

1. The project you are in charge of is a great success.

	PsG
A. *I kept a close watch over everyone's work.*	1
B. *Everyone devoted a lot of time and energy to it.*	0

2. You and your spouse (boyfriend/girlfriend) make up after a fight.

	PmG
A. *I forgave him/her.*	0
B. *I'm usually forgiving.*	1

3. You get lost driving to a friend's house.

	PsB
A. *I missed a turn.*	1
B. *My friend gave me bad directions.*	0

4. Your spouse (boyfriend/girlfriend) surprises you with a gift.

	PsG
A. *He/she just got a raise at work.*	0
B. *I took him/her out to a special dinner the night before.*	1

5. You forget your spouse's (boyfriend's/girlfriend's) birthday.

	PmB
A. *I'm not good at remembering birthdays.*	1
B. *I was preoccupied with other things.*	0

6. You get a flower from a secret admirer.

	PvG
A. *I am attractive to him/her.*	0
B. *I am a popular person.*	1

7. You run for a community office position and you win.

	PvG
A. *I devote a lot of time and energy to campaigning.*	0
B. *I work very hard at everything I do.*	1

8. You miss an important engagement.

	PvB
A. *Sometimes my memory fails me.*	1
B. *I sometimes forget to check my appointment book.*	0

9. You run for a community office position and you lose.

	PsB
A. *I didn't campaign hard enough.*	1
B. *The person who won knew more people.*	0

Figure 7.6 Test your optimism

10. You host a successful dinner.

	PmG
A. *I was particularly charming that night.*	0
B. *I am a good host.*	1

11. You stop a crime by calling the police.

	PsG
A. *A strange noise caught my attention.*	0
B. *I was alert that day.*	1

12. You were extremely healthy all year.

	PsG
A. *Few people around me were sick, so I wasn't exposed.*	0
B. *I made sure I ate well and got enough rest*	1

13. You owe the library ten dollars for an overdue book.

	PmB
A. *When I am really involved in what I am reading, I often forget when it's due.*	1
B. *I was so involved in writing the report that I forgot to return the book.*	0

14. Your stocks make you a lot of money.

	PmG
A. *My broker decided to take on something new.*	0
B. *My broker is a top-notch investor.*	1

15. You win an athletic contest.

	PmG
A. *I was feeling unbeatable.*	0
B. *I train hard.*	1

16. You fail an important examination.

	PsB
A. *I wasn't as smart as the other people taking the exam.*	1
B. *I didn't prepare for it well.*	0

17. You prepared a special meal for a friend and he/she barely touched the food.

	PvB
A. *I wasn't a good cook.*	1
B. *I made the meal in a rush.*	0

Figure 7.6   (continued)

18. You lose a sporting event for which you have been training for a long time.

	PvB
A. *I'm not very athletic.*	1
B. *I'm not good at that sport.*	0

19. Your car runs out of gas on a dark street late at night.

	PsB
A. *I didn't check to see how much gas was in the tank.*	1
B. *The gas gauge was broken.*	0

20. You lose your temper with a friend.

	PmB
A. *He/she is always nagging me.*	1
B. *He/she was in a hostile mood.*	0

21. You are penalized for not returning your income-tax forms on time.

	PmB
A. *I always put off doing my taxes.*	1
B. *I was lazy about getting my taxes done this year.*	0

22. You ask a person out on a date and he/she says no.

	PvB
A. *I was a wreck that day.*	1
B. *I got tongue-tied when I asked him/her on the date.*	0

23. A game-show host picks you out of the audience to participate in the show.

	PsG
A. *I was sitting in the right seat.*	0
B. *I looked the most enthusiastic.*	1

24. You are frequently asked to dance at a party.

	PmG
A. *I am outgoing at parties.*	1
B. *I was in perfect form that night.*	0

25. You buy your spouse (boyfriend/girlfriend) a gift and he/she doesn't like it.

	PsB
A. *I don't put enough thought into things like that.*	1
B. *He/she has very picky tastes.*	0

Figure 7.6 *(continued)*

26. You do exceptionally well in a job interview.

		PmG
A.	*I felt extremely confident during the interview.*	0
B.	*I interview well.*	1

27. You tell a joke and everyone laughs.

		PsG
A.	*The joke was funny.*	0
B.	*My timing was perfect.*	1

28. Your boss gives you too little time in which to finish a project, but you get it finished anyway.

		PvG
A.	*I am good at my job.*	0
B.	*I am an efficient person.*	1

29. You've been feeling run-down lately.

		PmB
A.	*I never get a chance to relax.*	1
B.	*I was exceptionally busy this week.*	0

30. You ask someone to dance and he/she says no.

		PsB
A.	*I am not a good enough dancer.*	1
B.	*He/she doesn't like to dance.*	0

31. You save a person from choking to death.

		PvG
A.	*I know a technique to stop someone from choking.*	0
B.	*I know what to do in crisis situations.*	1

32. Your romantic partner wants to cool things off for a while.

		PvB
A.	*I'm too self-centered.*	1
B.	*I don't spend enough time with him/her.*	0

33. A friend says something that hurts your feelings.

		PmB
A.	*She always blurts things out without thinking of others.*	1
B.	*My friend was in a bad mood and took it out on me.*	0

Figure 7.6   *(continued)*

34. Your employer comes to you for advice.

PvG

A. *I am an expert in the area about which I was asked.*   0
B. *I'm good at giving useful advice.*   1

35. A friend thanks you for helping him/her get through a bad time.

PvG

A. *I enjoy helping him/her through tough times.*   0
B. *I care about people.*   1

36. You have a wonderful time at a party.

PsG

A. *Everyone was friendly.*   0
B. *I was friendly.*   1

37. Your doctor tells you that you are in good physical shape.

PvG

A. *I make sure I exercise frequently.*   0
B. *I am very health-conscious.*   1

38. Your spouse (boyfriend/girlfriend) takes you away for a romantic weekend.

PmG

A. *He/she needed to get away for a few days.*   0
B. *He/she likes to explore new areas.*   1

39. Your doctor tells you that you eat too much sugar.

PsB

A. *I don't pay much attention to my diet.*   1
B. *You can't avoid sugar, it's in everything.*   0

40. You are asked to head an important project.

PmG

A. *I just successfully completed a similar project.*   0
B. *I am a good supervisor.*   1

41. You and your spouse (boyfriend/girlfriend) have been fighting a great deal.

PsB

A. *I have been feeling cranky and pressured lately.*   1
B. *He/she has been hostile lately.*   0

Figure 7.6 (continued)

42. You fall down a great deal while skiing.

PmB

A. *Skiing is difficult.*   1
B. *The trails were icy.*   0

43. You win a prestigious award.

PvG

A. *I solved an important problem.*   0
B. *I was the best employee.*   1

44. Your stocks are at an all-time low.

PvB

A. *I didn't know much about the business climate at the time.*   1
B. *I made a poor choice of stocks.*   0

45. You win the lottery.

PsG

A. *It was pure chance.*   0
B. *I picked the right numbers*   1

46. You gain weight over the holidays and you can't lose it.

PmB

A. *Diets don't work in the long run.*   1
B. *The diet I tried didn't work.*   0

47. You are in the hospital and few people come to visit.

PsB

A. *I'm irritable when I am sick.*   1
B. *My friends are negligent about things like that.*   0

48. They won't honor your credit card at a store.

PvB

A. *I sometimes overestimate how much money I have.*   1
B. *I sometimes forget to pay my credit-card bill.*   0

Scoring Key

PmB _____		PmG _____
PvB _____		PvG _____
	HoB _____	
PsB _____		PsG _____
Total B _____		Total G _____
	G–B _____	

Figure 7.6 *(continued)*

Interpreting Your Test

The test results will give you a clue as to your explanatory style, the ways in which you explain things to yourself. It tells you your habit of thought. Again, remember there are no right or wrong answers.

There are three crucial dimensions to your explanatory style: permanence, pervasiveness, and personalization. Each dimension, plus a couple of others, will be scored from your test.

Permanence   When pessimists are faced with challenges or bad events, they view these events as being permanent. In contrast, people who are optimists tend to view the challenges or bad events as temporary. Here are some statements that reflect some subtle differences:

Permanent (Pessimistic)	*Temporary (Optimistic)*
"My boss is a always a jerk."	"My boss is in a bad mood today."
"You never listen."	"You are not listening."
"This bad luck will never stop."	"My luck has got to turn."

To determine how you view bad events, look at the eight items in the test coded PmB (for Permanent Bad): 5, 13, 20, 21, 29, 33, 42, and 46. Those followed by 0 are optimistic, those followed by 1 are pessimistic. Total the numbers at the right-hand margin of the questions coded PmB and write the total on the PmB line on the scoring key.

If you totaled 0 or 1, you are very optimistic on this dimension; 2 or 3 is a moderately optimistic score; 4 is average; 5 or 6 is quite pessimistic; 7 or 8 is extremely pessimistic.

Now let's take a look at the difference in explanatory style between pessimists and optimists when there is a positive event in their lives. It's just the opposite of what happened with a bad event. Pessimists view positive events as temporary while optimists view them as permanent. Here again are some subtle difference in how pessimists and optimists might communicate their good fortune:

Temporary (Pessimistic)	Permanent (Optimistic)
"It's my lucky day."	"I am always lucky."
"My opponent was off today."	"I am getting better everyday."
"I tried hard today."	"I always give my best"

Now total all the questions coded PmG (for Permanent Good): 1, 10, 14, 15, 24, 26, 38, and 40. Write the total on the line in the scoring key marked PmG.

If you totaled 7 or 8, you are very optimistic on this dimension; 6 is a moderately optimistic score; 4 or 5 is average; 3 is pessimistic; 0, 1, or 2 is extremely pessimistic.

Are you starting to see a pattern? If you are scoring as a pessimist, you may want to learn how to be more optimistic. Your anxiety may be due to your belief that bad things are always going to happen, while good things are only a fluke.

Pervasiveness   This describes the tendency to perceive things either in universals (everyone, always, never) versus specifics (a specific individual, a specific time). Pessimists tend to describe things in universals while optimists use specifics.

Universal (Pessimists)	Specific (Optimist)
"All lawyers are jerks."	"My attorney was a jerk."
"Instruction manuals are worthless."	"This instruction manual is worthless."
"He is repulsive."	"He is repulsive to me."

Total your score for the questions coded PvB (for Pervasive Bad): 8, 16, 17, 18, 22, 32, 44, and 48. Write the total on the PvB line.

If you totaled 0 or 1, you are very optimistic on this dimension; 2 or 3 is a moderately optimistic score; 4 is average; 5 or 6 is quite pessimistic; 7 or 8 is extremely pessimistic.

Now let's look at the level of pervasiveness of good events. Optimists tend to view good events as universal, while pessimists view them as specific. Again, its just the opposite of how each views a bad event.

Total your score for the questions coded PvG (for Pervasive Good): 6, 7, 28, 31, 34, 35, 37, and 43. And write the total on the line labeled PvG.

If you totaled 7 or 8, you are very optimistic on this dimension; 6 is a moderately optimistic score; 4 or 5 is average; 3 is pessimistic; 0, 1 or 2 is extremely pessimistic.

Hope   The level of hope of hopelessness is determined by our combined level of permanence and pervasiveness. Your level of hope may be the most significant score for this test. Take your PvB and add it to your PmB score. This is your hope score.

If it is 0, 1, or 2, you are extraordinarily hopeful; 3, 4, 5, or 6 is a moderately hopeful score; 7 or 8 is average; 9, 10, or 11 is moderately hopeless; and 12, 13, 14, 15, or 16 is severely hopeless.

People who make permanent and universal explanations for their troubles tend to suffer from stress, anxiety, and depression and to collapse when things go bad. According to Dr. Seligman, no other score is as important as your hope score.

Personalization   When bad things happen we can either blame ourselves (internalize) and lower our self-esteem as a consequence or we can blame it on things beyond our control (externalize). Although it may not be right to deny personal responsibility, people who tend to externalize with bad events have higher self-esteem and are more optimistic.

Total your score for those questions coded PsB (for Personalization Bad): 3, 19, 19, 25, 30, 39, 41, and 47.

A score of 0 or 1 indicates very high self-esteem and optimism; 2 or 3 indicates moderate self-esteem; 4 is average; 5 or 6 indicates moderately low self esteem; and 7 or 8 indicates very low self-esteem.

Now let's take a look at personalization and good events. Again, the opposite occurs compared to bad events: When good things happen, the person with high self-esteem internalizes while the person with low self-esteem externalizes.

Total your score for those questions coded PsG (for Personalization Good): 1, 4, 11, 12, 23, 27, 36, and 45. Write your score on the line marked PsG on your scoring key.

If you totaled 7 or 8, you are very optimistic on this dimension; 6 is a moderately optimistic score; 4 or 5 is average; 3 is pessimistic; 0, 1 or 2 is extremely pessimistic.

Your Overall Scores   To compute your overall scores, first add the three B's (PmB + PvB + PsB). This is your B (Bad Event) score. Do the same for all of the G's (PmG + PvG + PsB). This is your G score. Subtract B from G to get your overall score.

If your B score is from 3 to 6, you are marvelously optimistic when bad events occur; 10 or 11 is average; 12 to 14 is pessimistic; anything above 14 is extremely pessimistic.

If your G score is 19 or above, you think about good events extremely optimistically; 14 to 16 is average; 11 to 13 indicates pessimism; and a score of 10 or less indicates great pessimism.

If your overall score (G minus B) is above 8, you are very optimistic across the board; 6 to 8, you are moderately optimistic; 3 to 5 is average; 1 or 2 is pessimistic; and a score of zero or below is very pessimistic.

Learning Optimism

It is important to learn how to be optimistic if you are a pessimist. Why? Studies have shown that optimists are healthier, happier, and enjoy life at a much higher level than pessimists. Learning to be optimistic means getting in the habit of thinking with a positive attitude. If you are pessimistic, it is probably because you have gotten into the habit of thinking in a negative framework.

According to Dr. Seligman, by far the world's leading authority on optimism, humans are by nature optimists. Nature has equipped us with an underlying optimism, because optimism is a necessary step towards achieving our goals in life. The first step in building an optimistic or positive mental attitude is taking personal responsibility for your own positive mental state, your life, your current situation, and your health. The next step is taking action to make the changes you desire.

I am going to provide some guidelines for conditioning your attitude for optimism, but I strongly encourage you to read other books that provide "blueprints" for optimism. In addition to Dr. Seligman's book *Learned Optimism*, a couple of other self-help books which I have found extremely helpful in my own life, as well as the lives of some patients, are the following:

The 7 Habits of Highly Effective People by Steven Covey (Simon and Schuster, New York, 1989)

Bringing Out the Best in People by Alan Loy McGinnis (Augsberg, Minneapolis, 1985)

Awaken the Giant Within by Anthony Robbins (Simon and Schuster, New York, 1991)

See You at the Top by Zig Zigler (Pelican Publishing, Gretna, LA, 1975)

In addition to reading these books, I recommend listening to motivational and/or relaxation tapes on a regular basis.

Conditioning Your Mind and Attitude

Achieving or maintaining high self-esteem and a healthy, positive mental attitude are critical factors to health. To achieve these states of mind you need to exercise or condition your attitude in much the same way you condition your body. Set attainable goals, write them down, and document your successes. Create and recite positive affirmations. Watch your self-talk, make sure that it supports your self-esteem.

One of the most powerful ways to improve the quality of your life is to improve the quality of your self-talk. According to Anthony Robbins, author of the bestsellers *Unlimited Power* and *Awaken the Giant Within,* the quality of your life is equal to the quality of the questions you habitually ask yourself. This is based on the belief that whatever question you ask your brain, you will get an answer.

Let's look at the following example: An individual is met with a particular challenge or problem. He or she can ask a number of questions in this situation. Questions some people may ask in this circumstance include: "Why does this always happen to me?" or, "Why am I always so stupid?" Do they get answers to these questions? Do the answers build self-esteem? Does the problem keep reappearing? What would be a higher quality question? How about, "This is a very interesting situation. What do I need to learn from this situation so that it never happens again?" Or, how about, "What can I do to make this situation better?"

In another example, let's look at individuals who suffer from depression. What are some questions they might ask themselves which may not be helping their situation? How about, "Why am I *always* so depressed? Why do things *always* seem to go wrong for me? Why am I so unhappy?" What are some better questions they may want to ask themselves? How about, "What do I need to do to gain more enjoyment and happiness in my life? What do I need to commit to in order to have more happiness and energy in my life?" After they have answered these questions, I have my depressed patients ask themselves, "If I had happiness and high energy levels right now, what would it feel like?" You will be amazed at how powerful questions can be in your life.

When your mind is searching for answers to these questions, it is reprogramming your subconscious into believing you have an abundance of energy. Unless there is a physiological reason for the chronic fatigue, it won't take long before your subconscious believes.

Regardless of the situation, asking better questions is bound to improve your attitude. If you want to have a better life, ask better questions. It sounds simple, because it is. If you want more energy, excitement, and happiness in your life, ask yourself the following questions on a consistent basis.

The Morning Questions

1. What am I most happy about in my life right now?
   Why does that make me happy?
   How does that make me feel?
2. What am I most excited about in my life right now?
   Why does that make me excited?
   How does that make me feel?
3. What am I most grateful about in my life right now?
   Why does that make me grateful?
   How does that make me feel?

4. What am I enjoying most about my life right now?
   What about that do I enjoy?
   How does that make me feel?
5. What am I committed to in my life right now?
   Why am I committed to that?
   How does that make me feel?
6. Who do I love? (starting close and moving out)
   Who loves me?
7. What must I do today to achieve my long-term goal?

The Evening Questions
1. What have I given today?
   In what ways have I been a giver today?
2. What did I learn today?
3. What did I do today to reach my long-term goal?
4. In what ways was today a perfect day?
5. Repeat morning questions.

Problem or Challenge Questions
1. What is right/great about this problem?
2. What is not perfect yet?
3. What am I willing to not do to make it the way I want?
4. How can I enjoy doing the things necessary to make it the way I want it?

Exercise to Beat Depression Naturally

Perhaps the most natural and certainly the safest antidepressant in the world is physical exercise. Often prescription drugs for elevating the mood are prescribed to be taken once or twice a day. How about a prescription for brisk walking for a half hour once or twice a day instead of a drug? The exercise itself enhances the most powerful mood elevators in the body, the endorphin system in the brain. As discussed in Chapter 5, a clear association exists between exercise and endorphin elevation; when endorphins go up, mood follows.

Chapter Summary

This chapter has provided some general guidelines in the natural treatment of anxiety. Foremost are the recommendations to avoid caffeine and substances which promote the conversion of pyruvate to lactic acid. While the current medical view of anxiety and depression has focused on biochemical models, the social and psychological model developed by Martin Seligman, Ph.D., may prove to be a better view. Learning to become more optimistic is critical to relieving anxiety and depression.

9

Natural Alternatives to Anti-Anxiety Drugs

The majority of the nearly 14 million Americans suffering from anxiety are given a prescription for tranquilizers (benzodiazepines) like Valium, Xanax, Halcion, Librium, Tranxene, Dalmane, and Klonopin, or perhaps an antidepressant like Prozac. These drugs are among the most widely prescribed even though their problems are well known. As pointed out previously, benzodiazepines are highly addictive and can cause impairment of mental function, drowsiness, lethargy, and many other possible side effects, while Prozac can cause bizarre irrational behavior, allergic reactions, headaches, nausea, and a number of other side effects.

Prescribing natural anxiolytic (anxiety-relieving) substances that could be just as effective in relieving the symptoms of anxiety as the benzodiazepines, but without the negative side effects, would be a major development in clinical practice. These natural substances exist. For example, the standardized extract of kava root and L.72 Anti-Anxiety (a homeopathic formula) have been shown to be as effective as drug therapy in relieving symptoms, and produce virtually no side effects. Another natural substance, GABA (gamma-aminobutyric acid) may also prove to be effective. And, if depression is the cause of the anxiety, an alternative to Prozac is the herb St. John's wort. Of all the natural substances, I feel kava is the most interesting and the most promising, so it will be discussed first and the most extensively.

Kava: Nature's Herbal Anxiolytic

The area of Oceania, the island communities of the Pacific including Micronesia, Melanesia, and Polynesia, is one of the few geographic areas of the world which did not have alcoholic beverages before European contact in the 18th century. However, these islanders did possess a magical drink used in ceremonies and celebrations because of its calming effect and ability to promote sociability. The drink, called kava, is still used today in this region of the world, a region where the people are often referred to as the happiest and friendliest in the world. Preparations of kava root (*Piper methysticum*) are now gaining greater popularity in Europe and the United States as mild sedatives and anxiolytics.

The History of Kava

The origins of kava usage are not known as it predates written history in Oceania.[1,2] It was first described for the western world by captain James Cook in the account of his voyage to the South Seas in 1768. Many myths and legends surround the early use of kava. The plant itself probably originated in the New Guinea–Indonesia area and was spread from island to island by early Polynesian explorers in canoes along with other plants. Each culture has its own story on the origins of kava. For example, in Samoa a story is told about the origins of kava and sugarcane. The story goes that a Samoan girl went to Fiji where she married a great chief. After some time, she returned to Samoa, but before doing so she noticed two plants growing on a hill. She saw a rat chewing on one of the plants and noticed the rat seemed to go to sleep. She concluded that the plant was a comforting food. She decided she would take this plant, sugarcane, back to Samoa, but then she noticed that the rat awoke and began to chew the root of another plant—kava. The animal who had been weak and shy became bold, strong, and more energetic. She decided that she would take both plants back with her to plant in Samoa. The plants grew very well in Samoa and soon a chief from a neighboring island exchanged two laying hens for roots of the two plants. Hence, the Samoans take credit for the spread of both the sugarcane and kava.

In Tonga, the legend is told that a great chief named Loau who lived on the island of Euaiki went to visit his servant Feva' anga. Feva' anga wanted to give a feast in the honor of the chief, but it was a time of great famine. In desperation he and his wife killed and cooked their only daughter to be served to the chief. However, Loau recognized the human flesh in the food when it was served and would not eat it. He instructed Feva' anga to plant the food in the ground and to bring him the plant that would spring forth. On receiving the mature plant, Loau instructed that a drink be prepared from it and consumed with due ceremony.

The Kava Ceremony

Regardless of exactly how kava originated, it has been used in ceremonies by the Oceanic people for thousands of years. There are three basic kava ceremonies: the full ceremony, enacted on every formal occasion; that performed at the meetings of village elders, chiefs, and nobles and for visiting chiefs and dignitaries; and the less formal kava circle common to social occasions.[1,2]

The first step in any kava ceremony was the preparation of the beverage. A description of the classic process was given in 1777 by George Forster, a young naturalist on James Cook's second Pacific voyage:

> Kava is made in the most disgustful manner that can be imagined, from the juice contained in the roots of a species of pepper-tree. This root is cut small, and the pieces chewed by several people, who spit the macerated mass into a bowl, where some water (milk) of coconuts is poured upon it. They then strain it through a quantity of fibres of coconuts, squeezing the chips, till all their juices mix with the coconut milk; and the whole liquor is decanted into another bowl. They swallow this nauseous stuff as fast as possible; and some old topers value themselves on being able to empty a great number of bowls.

As this traditional method of preparation became frowned upon or made illegal by colonial governments and missionaries, more "sanitary" methods of preparation involving grinding or grating took its place in many parts of Oceania.

The full kava ceremony reserved for very highly honored guests involves leading all of the guests to a platform. The ceremony begins with the arrival of a group of young men dressed in ceremonial attire and carrying a bowl of the kava drink and necessary utensils. The bowl is placed between the kava preparers and the visitors. The kava is placed in a cup by a specially selected individual who then turns and faces the visitor and delivers the beverage to the chief guest. The guest is instructed to hold the cup with both hands and drink from it. If the whole cup is drained without stopping, everyone says *a maca* (pronounced "a matha," meaning "it is empty") and claps three times with cupped hands. The cup bearer then returns to the kava bowl and proceeds to serve the person next in rank or importance.

Important people visiting Fiji and other islands of Oceania still participate in kava ceremonies. For example, during a 1992 presidential campaign visit to Hawaii, Hillary Clinton participated in a kava ceremony conducted by the Samoan community on Oahu.

The Effects of Drinking Kava

Kava drinkers relate a pleasant sense of tranquility and sociability upon consumption. Subjective reports given by scientists who have sampled kava themselves are relatively abundant. One of the first scientific studies on kava was performed by the noted pharmacologist Louis Lewin in 1886. A later description written in 1927 is described in *Kava, the Pacific Drug* (Yale University Press, New Haven, CT, 1992) as follows:

> When the mixture is not too strong, the subject attains a state of happy unconcern, well-being and contentment, free of physical or psychological excitement. At the beginning conversation comes in a gentle, easy flow and hearing and sight are honed, becoming able to perceive subtle shades of sound and vision. Kava soothes temperaments. The drinker never becomes angry, unpleasant, quarrelsome or noisy, as happens with alcohol. Both natives and whites consider kava as a means of easing moral discomfort. The drinker remains master of his conscious and his reason. When consumption is excessive, however, the limbs become

tired, the muscles seem no longer to respond to the orders and control of the mind, walking becomes slow and unsteady and the drinker looks partially inebriated. He feels the need to lie down. . . . He is overcome by somnolence and finally drifts off to sleep.

A more recent description is provided by researcher R.J. Gregory, who writes from his own experience:

Kava seizes one's mind. This is not a literal seizure, but something does change in the processes by which information enters, is retrieved, or leads to actions as a result. Thinking is certainly affected by the kava experience, but not in the same ways as are found from caffeine, nicotine, alcohol, or marijuana. I would personally characterize the changes I experienced as going from lineal processing of information to a greater sense of "being" and contentment with being. Memory seemed to be enhanced, whereas restriction of data inputs was strongly desired, especially with regard to disturbances of light, movements, noise and so on. Peace and quiet were very important to maintain the inner sense of serenity. My senses seemed to be unusually sharpened, so that even whispers seemed to be loud while loud noises were extremely unpleasant.

Drinking about half a coconut shell (100 to 150 milliliters) of certain varieties of kava is strong enough to put most people into a deep, dreamless sleep within 30 minutes. Unlike alcohol and other sedatives, kava does not produce any morning hangover. The kava drinker awakens having fully recovered normal physical and mental capacities.

Identification of Active Compounds

Identifying the active ingredients of kava has been a laborious process over the past 100 years.[1] Many experts now believe the pharmacological activities of kava are due mostly, if not entirely, to the presence of compounds known as kavalactones (also referred to as kava alpha-pyrones). These compounds are found in the fat-soluble portion of the root. Although the kavalactones are the primary active components, other components appear to contribute to the sedative and anxiolytic activities of kava. In one study the sedative activity of a crude preparation was more effective than the isolated kavalactones. The kavalactone content of the root can vary between 3% and 20%, therefore, for clinical use, preparations standardized for kavalactone content are preferred to crude preparations.

Pharmacological Activity of Kavalactones

A team of scientists from the Freiburg University Institute of Pharmacology in Germany, led by Hans J. Meyer, conducted many of the first comprehensive studies on the activities of kavalactones in the 1950s and 1960s. Altogether, this research has determined that kavalactones exhibit sedative, analgesic, anticonvulsant, and muscle-relaxant effects in laboratory animals. These studies seemed to confirm the empirical and subjective observations.

More recent studies including those studies conducted by Dana D. Jamieson and colleagues at the University of New South Wales have confirmed and/or elaborated on these effects. Most notable are studies demonstrating that kavalactones exert many of their effects by non-traditional mechanisms. For example, most sedative drugs including the benzodiazepines (like Valium) work by binding to specific receptors (benzodiazepine or GABA receptors) in the brain which then leads to chemical changes (potentiation of GABA effects) which promote sedation. Studies in animals have shown that the kavalactones do not bind to benzodiazepine or GABA receptors.[4] Instead, the kavalactones are thought to somehow modify receptor domains rather than interacting specifically with receptor-binding sites. Other studies have indicated that the kavalactones appear to act primarily on the limbic system—the ancient part of the brain which effects all other brain activities and is the principle seat of the emotions.[5] It is thought that kava may also promote sleep by altering the way in which the limbic system modulates emotional processes. It also appears that many of the laboratory models of identifying how a substance works to promote a calming effect are simply not sophisticated enough to evaluate the kavalactones.

In another example of the uncharacteristic pharmacological qualities of kava, a study designed to evaluate its pain-relieving effects could not demonstrate any binding to opiate receptors.[6] The significance of this finding is that the study used some models where non-opiate analgesics like aspirin and other non-steroidal anti-inflammatory drugs are ineffective. In addition, it was determined that the sedative or muscle-relaxing effects were not responsible for the pain-relieving effects. What all of these findings mean is that kava reduces pain in a manner unlike morphine, aspirin, or any other pain reliever.

An interesting effect of kava compared to many anxiolytic drugs is that unlike the drugs, kava does not lose effectiveness with time. Loss of effectiveness of a drug is known as "tolerance." Kavalactones, even when administered in huge amounts, demonstrated absolutely no loss of effectiveness in animal studies.[7] This is another example of the uncharacteristic qualities of kava.

Another pharmacological activity of kava worth mentioning is its ability to protect against brain damage due to ischemia.[8] This effect has been demonstrated in two animal models of focal cerebral ischemia. The effectiveness of the kavalactones was due to their ability to limit the infarct area as well as a mild anticonvulsant effect. Kava extract may prove useful in recovery from stroke.

Clinical Studies with Kava Extracts

Several European countries have approved kava preparations in the treatment of nervous anxiety, insomnia, and restlessness on the basis of detailed pharmacological data and favorable clinical studies.

Earlier clinical trials used D,L-kavain, a purified kavalactone, at a dose of 400 milligrams per day. For example, in one double-blind placebo-controlled study of 84 patients with anxiety symptoms, kavain was shown to improve vigilance, memory, and reaction time.[9] In another double-blind study, kavain was compared to the drug oxazepam (a drug similar to diazepam or Valium) in 38 patients.[10] Both substances caused progressive improvements in two different anxiety scores (Anxiety Status Inventory and the Self-Rating Anxiety Scale) over a four-week period. However, while oxazepam and similar drugs are associated with being addictive as well as with side effects, kavain appeared free of these complications.

More recent studies have featured well-defined kava extracts. As mentioned earlier, evidence suggests that the whole complex of kavalactones and other compounds naturally found in kava produce greater pharmacological activity. In addition, studies have shown that kavalactones are more rapidly absorbed when given orally as an extract of the root rather than the isolated kavalactones. The bioavailability of lactones, as measured by peak plasma concentrations, is up to three to five times higher from the extract than when given as isolated substances.[3] Further evidence that kava root extracts are superior to isolated kavalactones is offered by an animal study showing that while isolated kavalactones are taken up into brain tissue at a good level, when a crude kava preparation was given the concentrations of lactones was 2 to 20 times higher.[11] From this evidence it appears that crude extracts standardized for kavalactone content may offer the greatest therapeutic benefit.

Several clinical trials have featured a special kava extract standardized to contain 70% kavalactones; however, this high percentage of kavalactones may be sacrificing some of the other constituents that may contribute to the pharmacology of kava. Therefore, preparations around 30% may prove to be the most ideal. More important than the actual percentage of kavalactones is the total dosage of the kavalactones and the assurance that the full-range of kavalactones are present.

In perhaps the most significant study, a 70% kavalactone extract was shown to exhibit significant therapeutic benefit in patients suffering from anxiety.[12] The study was double-blind; 29 patients were assigned to receive 100 milligrams of the kava extract three times daily while another 29 patients received a placebo. Therapeutic effectiveness was assessed using several standard psychological assessments including the Hamilton Anxiety Scale. The result of this four-week study indicated that individuals taking the kava extract had a statistically significant reduction in symptoms of anxiety, including feelings of nervousness and somatic complaints such as heart palpitations, chest pains, headache, dizziness, and feelings of gastric irritation. No side effects were reported with the kava extract.

In another double-blind study, two groups of 20 women with menopause-related symptoms were treated for a period of eight weeks with the 70% kavalactone extract (100 milligrams, three times daily) or placebo.[13] The target variable was once again the Hamilton Anxiety Scale. The group receiving the kava extract demonstrated significant improvement at the end of the very first week of treatment.

Scores continued to improve over the course of the eight-week study. In addition to improvement in symptoms of stress and anxiety, a number of other symptoms also improved. Most notably there was an overall improvement in subjective well-being, mood, and general symptoms of menopause including hot flashes. Again no side effects were noted.

Two additional studies have shown that unlike benzo-diazepines, alcohol, and other drugs, kava extract is not associated with depressed mental function or impairment in driving or the operation of heavy equipment.[14,15] In one of these studies 12 healthy volunteers were tested in a double-blind crossover manner to assess the effects of oxazepam (placebo on days one to three, 15 milligrams on the day before testing, 75 milligrams on the morning of the experiment), the extract of kava standardized at 70% kavalactones (200 milligrams, three times daily for five days), and a placebo on behavior and event-related potentials (ERPs) in electroencephalograph (EEG) readings in a recognition/memory task. The subjects' task was to identify within a list of visually presented words those that were shown for the first time and those that were being repeated. Consistent with other benzodiazepines, oxazepam inhibited the recognition of both new and old words as noted by ERP. In contrast, kava showed a slightly increased recognition rate and a larger ERP difference between old and new words. The results of this study once again demonstrate the uncharacteristic effects of kava; in this case, it improves anxiety, but unlike standard anxiolytics, kava actually improves mental function, and at the recommended levels does not promote sedation.

Dosage of Kava The dosage of kava preparations is based on the level of kavalactones. Based on clinical studies using pure kavalactones or kava extracts standardized for kavalactones, the recommendation for anxiolytic effects is 45 to 70 milligrams of kavalactones three times daily. For sedative effects, the same daily quantity (135 to 210 milligrams) can be taken as a single dose one hour before retiring.

To put the therapeutic dosage in perspective it is important to point out that a standard bowl of traditionally prepared kava drink contains approximately 250 milligrams of kavalactones and several bowls may be consumed at one sitting.

Toxicology of Kava   Although no side effects have been reported using standardized kava extracts at recommended levels, it is possible that side effects may be present at high dosages. High dosages of kava beverages consumed daily over a prolonged period (a few months to a year or more) are associated with "kava dermopathy"—a condition of the skin characterized by a peculiar generalized scaly eruption known as kani.[16] The skin becomes dry and covered with scales, especially the palms of the hand, soles of the feet, forearms, the back, and shins. It was thought at one time that kava dermopathy may be due to interference with niacin. However, in a double-blind placebo-controlled study no therapeutic effect with niacinamide (100 milligrams daily) could be demonstrated.[17] It appears the only effective treatment for kava dermopathy is reduction or cessation of kava consumption. Again, no reported cases of kava dermopathy have been noted in individuals taking standardized kava extracts at recommended levels.

Other adverse effects of extremely high doses of kava (greater than 310 grams per week) for prolonged periods include biochemical abnormalities (low levels of serum albumin, protein, urea, and bilirubin), presence of blood in the urine, increased red blood cell volume, decreased platelet and lymphocyte counts, and shortness of breath.[18] The presence of these adverse effects are questionable because the subjects also reported heavy alcohol and cigarette usage. Nonetheless, high doses of kava are unnecessary and should not be encouraged.

L.72 Anti-Anxiety: Natural Anxiolytic

A special homeopathic combination—L.72 Anti-Anxiety—has also been shown to be as effective as diazepam (Valium) in a randomized trial.[19] If you are not familiar with homeopathy, it is a two-hundred-year-old system of medicine where symptoms are treated with minute quantities of drugs (usually herbs) that would normally bring on those very same symptoms.

The word homeopathy comes from the Greek word *homoios*, which means like, and *pathos*, which means suffering. Homeopathy is based on the principle that "like cures like." In other words, a substance that can cause a symptom in a healthy person may treat the same symptom in a sick person. Homeopathy was extremely popular in the United States at the turn of the 19th century, but as the drug companies rose in prominence, they effectively suppressed this form of medicine. Homeopathy remained popular in many parts of the world, especially Europe and India, and is now experiencing a tremendous rise in popularity in the United States. If you would like more information on this form of medicine contact the Homeopathic Educational Services, 2124 Kittredge St., Berkeley, CA 94704, (510) 649-0294. They have an impressive catalog. If you are looking for a good book on homeopathy, I recommend any of the many books on the subject written by Dana Ullman.

L.72 Anti-Anxiety formula is manufactured by Lehning Laboratories, one of the leading manufacturers of homeopathic medicines in France, and distributed in the United States by Enzymatic Therapy. L.72 is composed of the following homeopathic medicines: *Cicuta virosa* 4X, *Ignatia* 4X, *Staphysagria* 4X, *Asfoetida* 3X, *Corydalis formosa* 3X, *Sumbulus moschatus* 3X, *Olei gaultheria procubens* 4X, *Valeriana officinalis* 3X, *Hyoscyamus* 3X, and *Avena sativa* 1X.

As mentioned earlier, L.72 was shown to be as effective as diazepam (Valium) in a randomized trial.[19] In the study, 30 women received L.72 and 30 women received 2 milligrams of diazepam. The patients were evaluated before and after a 30-day treatment with the aid of a special scoring scale, known as the Hamilton scale, that is often used to evaluate anxiety. The results indicated that L.72 was as effective as diazepam in reducing anxiety, phobia, and emotional instability. The same held true for symptoms that often accompany anxiety: hot flashes, rapid heartbeat, shortness of breath, intestinal problems, frequent urination, and dizziness.

A spectacular gain in the number of hours of sleep and a considerable decrease in pulse rate were noted in both groups; however, the women receiving the L.72 demonstrated a better overall response. On day one, patients using L.72 had an average pulse rate of 93. At the end of the 30-day study, this had been reduced to 83.

The overall assessment of the patients and physicians who participated in the study was that L.72 was as effective as diazepam in reducing symptoms of anxiety and depression. The big difference, however, is that while diazepam is associated with significant toxicity and addiction, L.72 is without side effects and is non-addictive. It is also much less expensive. Take L.72 Anti-Anxiety formula by placing 20 drops in 2 to 3 ounces of water, three to four times per day.

GABA

Benzodiazepine drugs like Valium work by stimulating receptors in the brain for gamma-aminobutyric acid (GABA)—the brain's natural calming agent. Although GABA is manufactured from the amino acid glutamine in the brain, in some cases of anxiety, panic disorders, and depression the brain does not make enough GABA.

Although to my knowledge there are no clinical trials of GABA in anxiety, GABA has been used with reported success at the famed Princeton Brain Bio Center.[20] Eric Braverman, M.D., and Carl Pfeiffer, M.D., reported in their book *The Healing Nutrients Within: Facts, Findings, and New Research on Amino Acids* (Keats Publishing, New Canaan, CT, 1987) that GABA has been used in a variety of brain disorders including epilepsy and schizophrenia. For anxiety, these experts recommend that GABA be used in severely anxious individuals addicted to benzodiazepines at a dosage of 200 milligrams four times daily.

St. John's Wort

Perhaps the best herbal supprt to use if anxiety is due primarily to depression is St. John's wort (*Hypericum perforatum*), a shrubby perennial plant native to many parts of the world including Europe and the United States. Researchers in Germany have discovered components in St. John's wort that alter brain chemistry in a way that improves mood. In one study, six women with depressive symptoms, ages 55 and 65, were given a standardized extract of St. John's wort (0.125% hypericin) as the only therapy.[21] There was a significant increase in urinary metabolites of the important brain chemical dopamine, indicating that there was greater dopamine production in the brain, which is consistent with antidepressant effects of many drugs. In addition, when these six patients and an additional nine cases were evaluated with surveys that measure anxiety, mood disturbances, loss of interest, hypersomnia, anorexia, depression, psychomotor retardation and feelings of worthlessness, the rating was significantly lower than the same ratings prior to taking the herb.

Other clinical studies showed the standardized extract of St. John's wort to be more effective in relieving depression than several standard drugs often prescribed for depression including amitriptyline (Elavil) and imiprimine

(Trofinil).[22] While these drugs are associated with significant side effects (most often drowsiness, dry mouth, constipation, and impaired urination), St. John's wort extract is not associated with any significant side effects. In addition to improving mood, the extract has been shown to greatly improve sleep quality; it was effective in relieving both insomnia and hypersomnia.

The dosage of St. John's wort used in these German studies has typically been 300 milligrams of the extract (0.125% hypericin content) three times daily. If you want to experience the same level of benefit as that noted, be sure and use sources of St. John's wort standardized for hypericin.

Some Practical Advice

If you are suffering from anxiety you have some choices. My recommendation is to start off with the kava extract. Based on the clinical research, this should provide ample support as you work your way to a more positive, optimistic, and relaxed mental outlook. The L.72 Anti-Anxiety and GABA can be used in conjunction with the kava. In fact, I would recommend this combined approach for individuals with a history of either benzodiazepine or antidepressant therapy.

I would use the St. John's wort extract if depression is the primary condition, not anxiety.

Note: If you are currently on a tranquilizer or anti-depressant, you will need to work with a physician to get off the drug. Stopping the drug on your own can be dangerous; you absolutely must have proper medical supervision.

Chapter Summary

Over 14 million Americans suffer from anxiety. As a result prescriptions for benzodiazepines are extremely high, even though these drugs are associated with numerous problems including the fact that they are highly addictive. Two natural anxiolytic substances—standardized kava root extract and L.72 Anti-Anxiety—are as effective as standard drug therapy for anxiety, and free from the common side effects. Kava extract and L.72 can be used safely as natural alternatives to benzodiazepines in clinical practice.

Insomnia

10

The Natural Approach to Insomnia

Over the course of a year, over one-half of the U.S. population will have difficulty falling asleep. About 33% of the population experiences insomnia on a regular basis. Many use over-the-counter sedative medications to combat insomnia, while others seek stronger drugs. Each year up to 10 million people in the U.S. receive prescriptions for drugs to help them go to sleep.

Insomnia can have many causes, but the most common reasons are depression, anxiety, and tension. If psychological factors do not seem to be the cause, various foods, drinks, and medications may be responsible. There are numerous compounds in food and drink and well over 300 drugs which can interfere with normal sleep.

Common Causes of Insomnia
Anxiety or tension
Depression
Environmental change

Emotional arousal
Fear of insomnia
Fear of sleep
Nocturnal myoclonus
Hypoglycemia
Disruptive environment
Pain or discomfort
Caffeine
Drugs
Alcohol

Sedative Medications

The two primary classes of drugs used in the treatment of insomnia are antihistamines and benzodiazepines. The benzodiazepine drugs are available only by prescription. These drugs have been described in Chapter 7. Antihistamines are available in over-the-counter sleeping pills and contain either diphenhydramine or doxylamine. Antihistamines act to prevent the manufacture of histamine in the brain. This produces drowsiness and sleep.

Over-the-Counter Sedatives

Diphenhydramine	*Doxylamine*
Benadryl	Doxysom
Compoz	Ultra Sleep
Nervine	Unisom
Nytol	
Sleep-Eze 3	
Sleepinal	
Sominex	
Twilite	

Side Effects of Sleeping Pills

Drowsiness is the primary side effect with most antihistamines, especially those without stimulants. The warning on the product not to drive or operate heavy machinery should be taken quite seriously. As little as 50 milligrams of diphenhydramine (Benadryl) may produce an impairment in driving similar to a 0.1% blood alcohol content, the standard for drunk driving.[1] Other possible side effects include allergic reactions, headache, nausea, and drying of the nose, mouth, and throat.

The side effects of benzodiazepines have been previously discussed (see page 94).

The Vicious Cycle

While both antihistamines and benzodiazepines are effective in the short term, they cause significant problems in the long term. Benzodiazepines, in particular, are not designed to be used long-term, as they are addictive, associated with numerous side effects, and cause abnormal sleep patterns. Antihistamines also interfere with normal sleep patterns. As a result, people taking sleeping pills enter a viscious cycle. They take the drug to induce sleep which, in turn, causes further disruption of normal sleep. In the morning, in an attempt to "get going," they will typically drink large quantities of coffee.

Sleeping pills inhibit normal sleep and cause a morning hangover because they suppress REM (rapid eye movement) sleep. During REM sleep the body is more physiologically active; repair and rejuvenative processes take place. During REM sleep is when we dream. Because patients do not experience adequate REM sleep while on a benzodiazepine, they will typically wake up with a "hangover" and often feel more tired than when they went to sleep. When an individual tries to withdraw from long-term use of benzodiazepines, REM sleep is increased leading to nightmares and further sleep disturbances among other withdrawal symptoms.

Benzodiazepines, especially Halcion, have been receiving a great deal of negative attention in the media the past few years. More people are "waking up" to the fact, that these drugs can be quite dangerous if used for other than occasional use. If you have taken a benzodiazepine for more than four weeks, do not stop taking the drug suddenly. It is important to work with your physician to taper off the drug gradually to avoid potentially dangerous withdrawal symptoms. Symptoms of withdrawal can include anxiety, irritability, sensations of panic, insomnia, nausea, headache, impaired concentration, memory loss, depression, extreme sensitivity to the environment, seizures, hallucinations, and paranoia.

Dietary and Lifestyle Factors

Several dietary and lifestyle factors should be considered in relieving insomnia: elimination of food and drink compounds that impair sleep processes, avoiding nocturnal hypoglycemia, learning to relax, and exercise. Each of these factors are discussed below.

Elimination of Inhibitors of Sleep

It is essential that the diet be free of natural stimulants such as caffeine and related compounds. Coffee and less obvious caffeine sources such as soft drinks, chocolate, coffee-flavored ice cream, hot cocoa, and tea must all be eliminated.

Sensitivity to the stimulant effects of caffeine is extremely variable from one person to the next. This is largely a reflection of how quickly the body can eliminate caffeine. In other words, some people are more sensitive to the effects of caffeine than other people due to a slower elimination of these substances from the body. Even small amounts of caffeine such as those found in decaffeinated coffee or chocolate may be enough to cause insomnia in some people. (For more information on the stimulatory effects of caffeine and dietary sources see page 29.)

Another substance to eliminate is alcohol. Alcohol produces a number of effects that impair sleep. In addition to causing the release of adrenaline, alcohol impairs the transport of the amino acid tryptophan into the brain. The significance of this inhibition is that tryptophan is converted in the brain to serotonin, a natural sleep-promoting substance.

Nocturnal Hypoglycemia

Nocturnal hypoglycemia (low nighttime blood glucose level) is an important cause of sleep-maintenance insomnia. When there is a drop in the blood glucose level it causes the release of the hormones that regulate glucose levels, such as adrenaline, glucagon, cortisol, and the growth hormone. These compounds are stimulatory to the brain. They are a natural signal that it is time to eat.

Many people in the United States suffer from faulty glucose metabolism, either hypoglycemia or diabetes, because of overeating refined carbohydrates. The dietary guidelines given in Chapter 4 are important to follow to prevent nocturnal hypoglycemia.

Good bedtime snacks to keep blood sugar levels steady throughout the night are oatmeal and other whole grain cereals, whole grain breads and muffins, and other complex carbohydrates. These foods will not only help keep blood sugar levels appropriate, they actually help promote sleep by increasing the level of the natural sleep-promoting substance, serotonin, within the brain.

Progressive Relaxation

The progressive relaxation technique described in Chapter 3 can be quite effective in promoting relaxation and sleep. In the treatment of insomnia, continue to perform the progressive relaxation technique until it produces sleep.

Exercise

Regular physical exercise is known to improve general well-being as well as promote improvement in sleep quality. Exercise should be performed in the morning or early evening, not before bedtime, and should be of moderate intensity. Usually 20 minutes of aerobic exercise at a heart rate between 60% and 70% percent of maximum (approximately 220 minus age in years) is sufficient. (See Chapter 5 for additional information on how to design an exercise program.)

Natural Alternatives to Sedative Medications

Foremost in the natural approach to insomnia is the elimination of those factors known to disrupt normal sleep patterns such as sources of caffeine, alcohol, and drugs. Since insomnia is largely due to psychological factors, these should be considered and handled before simply inducing sleep with drugs. Counseling and/or stress reduction techniques such as progressive relaxation and exercise are often very effective. If these general measures produce no improvement, several natural alternatives to sedative medications can be used. In addition to kava (see pages 128–138), valerian is another herb that can be tried. Once a normal sleep pattern has been established, kava or valerian use should be slowly decreased.

Valerian

Valerian (*Valeriana officinalis*) has been widely used in folk medicine as a sedative. Recent scientific studies have substantiated valerian's ability to improve sleep quality and relieve insomnia.[2-4] In a large double-blind study involving 128 subjects it was shown that an aqueous extract of valerian root improved the subjective ratings for sleep quality and sleep latency (the time required to get to sleep) but left no "hangover" the next morning.[2]

In a followup study, valerian extract was shown to significantly reduce sleep latency and improve sleep quality in sufferers of insomnia under laboratory conditions and was suggested to be as effective in reducing sleep latency as small doses of benzodiazepines.[3] The difference, however, arises in the fact that these compounds also result in increased morning sleepiness. Valerian, on the other hand, actually reduces morning sleepiness.

As a mild sedative, valerian may be taken at the following dose 30 to 45 minutes before retiring:

Dried root (or as tea)	1 to 2 grams
Tincture (1:5)	4 to 6 milliliters (1 to 1.5 teaspoons)
Fluid extract (1:1)	1 to 2 milliliters (0.5 to 1 teaspoon)
Valerian extract (0.8% valeric acid)	150 to 300 milligrams

If morning sleepiness does occur, reduce dosage. If dosage was not effective, be sure to eliminate those factors that disrupt sleep such as caffeine and alcohol before increasing dosage.

Tryptophan

The amino acid tryptophan is converted in the brain to serotonin, a transmitting compound that is an important initiator of sleep. Since the synthesis of serotonin within the brain is dependent on the availability of the amino acid tryptophan, supplementing the diet with tryptophan produces very good results in relieving insomnia. Tryptophan administration at a dose of 1 to 3 grams has been shown to reduce the time required to go to sleep as well as decrease awakenings in numerous double-blind clinical studies.[5-7]

Unfortunately, at the time of this writing, tryptophan is no longer available to American consumers. For several decades, L-tryptophan was used by thousands of people in the United States safely and effectively for insomnia and depression. But in October 1989, some people taking tryptophan started reporting strange symptoms to physicians— severe muscle and joint pain, high fever, weakness, swelling of the arms and legs, and shortness of breath. The syndrome was dubbed EMS (eosinophilia-myalgia syndrome). This led to the removal of all products containing more than 100 milligrams of L-tryptophan from the market on November 17, 1989. As of May 1992, the number of reported EMS cases was 1,541 including 38 deaths.

All cases of tryptophan-induced EMS could be traced to one manufacturer, Showa Denko. Of the six Japanese companies supplying tryptophan to the United States, Showa Denko was the largest in that it supplied 50% to 60% of all the tryptophan being used. Due to a change in manufacturing procedures, Showa Denko's tryptophan produced from October 1988 to June 1989 became contaminated with a substance now linked to EMS.[8]

Tryptophan has remained off the market despite the fact that, before the Showa Denko incident, it had been used safely for decades. There are numerous examples of contaminated foods and medicines causing health problems and even death, yet, once the problem of contamination is solved, manufacturers are once again allowed to market their products, whether they are contaminated grapes, Perrier, or hamburgers from Jack in the Box. But, for some reason, tryptophan has not been allowed back in the marketplace even though the contamination issue has been solved. Hopefully, tryptophan will become available again in the very near future. It is interesting to note that one of the best treatments for EMS is non-contaminated tryptophan.[9]

The Restless Legs Syndrome

The restless legs syndrome is another significant cause of insomnia. This syndrome is characterized by an irresistible urge to move the legs while trying to sleep and while awake. Although the restless leg syndrome (RLS) is most often found in people consuming too much caffeine, some patients with restless legs syndrome respond well to extremely high doses of folic acid (35 to 60 milligrams daily).[10] This syndrome is believed to be a result of a folic acid deficiency or perhaps an increased need for folic acid in some individuals.

Another potential cause of RLS is low iron levels or low levels of the iron-binding protein in the blood known as ferritin. Low serum iron or ferritin levels have been found in psychiatric patients experiencing a condition called akathisia, coming from the Greek word meaning "can't sit down." Akathisia is a drug-induced state of agitation. The most common drugs producing akathisia are neuroleptics and Prozac. Several studies have shown that the level of iron depletion correlates with the severity of akathisia.

What prompted the research into iron status and akathisia was the association between low iron levels and the so-called restless legs syndrome (RLS) documented in clinical studies more than 30 years ago. However, while more recent studies have focused on low iron levels and akathisia, there has been little (if any) research on iron levels and RLS in the last few decades. This gap in research prompted researchers at the Department of Geriatric Medicine of the Royal Liverpool University in Liverpool, U.K., to study the relationship between iron status and RLS in 18 elderly patients and 18 controls.[11]

Serum ferritin levels were reduced in the RLS patients compared with controls; serum iron, vitamin B12, folic acid, and hemoglobin levels did not differ between the two groups. A rating scale with a maximum score of 10 was used to assess the severity of RLS symptoms. Serum ferritin levels were inversely correlated with the severity of RLS symptoms. Fifteen patients with RLS were treated with ferrous sulfate (200 milligrams, three times daily) for two months. The RLS severity score improved by a median of 4 points in six patients with an initial ferritin less than 18 micrograms per liter, by 3 points in four patients with ferritin levels between 18 and 45 micrograms per liter, and by 1 point in five patients with ferritin levels between 45 and 100 micrograms per liter.

The conclusion of the study: "Iron deficiency, with or without anemia, is an important contributor to the development of RLS in elderly patients, and iron supplements can produce a significant reduction in symptoms."

Almost all patients with restless legs syndrome also experience nocturnal myoclonus, a nerve and muscular disorder characterized by repeated contractions of one or more muscle groups, typically of the legs, during sleep. Each jerk usually lasts less than 10 seconds. The person with nocturnal myoclonus is normally unaware of the myoclonus and only complains of either frequent nocturnal awakenings or excessive daytime sleepiness. But questioning the sleep partner often reveals the myoclonus. Vitamin E may be helpful in relieving nocturnal myoclonus. Take at least 800 IU per day.

Chapter Summary

Insomnia is an extremely common problem in the United States. While most people choose to take over-the-counter or prescription sedatives, addressing the underlying factors contributing to the insomnia and the use of natural sedatives like kava and valerian appears to be a safer and more effective approach in the long term. If an individual suffers from the restless legs syndrome, folic acid and/or iron therapy may be effective. For nocturnal myoclonus, give vitamin E a try.

References

Chapter 1: What Is Stress?

1. Holmes TH and Rahe RH: The social readjustment scale. J Psychosom Res 11:213–8, 1967.
2. Seyle H: Stress and Life. McGraw-Hill, New York, 1976.

Chapter 2: Comprehensive Stress Management

1. Beasley JD: The Betrayal of Health: The Impact of Nutrition, Environment, and Lifestyle on Illness in America. Times Books, New York, 1991.

Chapter 3: Calming the Mind and Body

1. Benson H: The Relaxation Response. William Morrow, New York, 1975.

Chapter 4: Dietary Guidelines

1. Lee MA, et al.: Anxiety and caffeine consumption in people with anxiety disorders. Psychiatr Res 15:211–7, 1985.

2. Chou T. Wake up and smell the coffee: Caffeine, coffee, and the medical consequences. West J Med 157:544–53, 1992.

3. Hughes JR, et al.: Caffeine self-administration, withdrawal, and adverse effects among coffee drinkers. Arch Gen Psych 48:611–7, 1991.

4. Estler CJ, Ammon HP and Herzog C: Swimming capacity of mice after prolonged treatment with psychostimulants. I. Effects of caffeine on swimming performance and cold stress. Psychopharmaco 58:161–6, 1978.

5. Greden JF, et al.: Anxiety and depression associated with caffeinism among psychiatric inpatients. Am J Psychiatry 135:963–6, 1978.

6. Montiero MG, et al.: Subjective feelings of anxiety in young men after ethanol and diazepam infusions. J Clin Psychiatry 51:12–6, 1990.

7. Winokur A, et al.: Insulin resistance after glucose tolerance testing in patients with major depression. Am J Psychiatry 145:325–30, 1988.

8. Wright JH, et al.: Glucose metabolism in unipolar depression. Br J Psychiatry 132:386–93, 1978.

9. Jenkins DJA, et al.: Glycemic index of foods: A physiological basis for carbohydrate serving. Am J Clin Nutr 24:362–6, 1981.

10. Truswell AS: Glycemic index of foods. Eur J Clin Nutr 46 (Supplement 2):S91–101, 1992.

11. Rowe AH and Rowe A, Jr.: Food Allergy: Its Manifestations and Control and the Elimination Diets: A Compendium. Charles C. Thomas, Springfield, IL, 1972.

12. Breneman JC: Basics of Food Allergy. Charles C. Thomas, Springfield, IL, 1977.

13. Brostoff J and Challacombe SJ (eds): Food Allergy and Intolerance. WB Saunders, Philadelphia, 1987.

Chapter 5: Exercise and Stress Reduction

1. Pollack ML, Wilmore JH, and Fox SM: Exercise in Health and Disease. WB Saunders, Philadelphia, 1984.
2. Farmer ME, et al.: Physical activity and depressive symptomatology: The NHANES 1 epidemiologic follow-up study. Am J Epidemiol 1328:1340–51, 1988.
3. Daniel Carr, et al.: Physical conditioning facilitates the exercised-induced secretion of beta-endorphin and beta-lipoprotein in women. New Engl J Med 305:560–5, 1981.
4. Lobstein D, Mosbacher BJ, and Ismail AH: Depression as a powerful discriminator between physically active and sedentary middle-aged men. J Psychosom Res 27:69–76, 1983.

Chapter 6: Nutritional and Herbal Support

1. Block G, et al.: Vitamin supplement use, by demographic characteristics. Amer J Epidemiol 127:297–309, 1988.
2. National Research Council: Diet and Health. Implications for Reducing Chronic Disease Risk. National Academy Press, Washington, D.C., 1989.
3. National Research Council: Recommended Dietary Allowances, 10th edition. National Academy Press, Washington, D.C., 1989.
4. Cheraskin E: Vitamin C—Who Needs It? Arlington Press, Birmingham, AL, 1993.
5. Shils ME and Young VR: Modern Nutrition in Health and Disease, 7th edition. Lea and Febiger, Philadelphia, 1988.
6. Farnsworth NR, et al.: Siberian ginseng (*Eleutherococcus senticosus*): Current status as an adaptogen. Econ Med Plant Res 1:156–215, 1985.
7. Hikino H: Traditional remedies and modern assessment: The case of ginseng. In: The Medicinal Plant Industry. Wijeskera ROB (ed). CRC Press, Boca Raton, FL, 1991, Chapter 11, pp. 149–66.
8. Shibata S, et al.: Chemistry and pharmacology of Panax. Econ Med Plant Res 1:217–84, 1985.

9. Hallstrom C, Fulder S, and Carruthers M: Effect of ginseng on the performance of nurses on night duty. Comp Med East and West 6:277–82, 1982.

10. Bhattacharya SK and Mitra SK: Anxiolytic activity of Panax ginseng roots: An experimental study. J Ethnopharmacol 34:87–92, 1991.

11. Britton SW and Silvette H: Further experiments on cortico-adrenal extract: Its efficacy by mouth. Science 74:440–1, 1931.

Chapter 7: Understanding Anxiety

1. Eaton WW, et al.: Panic and panic disorder in the United States. Am J Psychiatry 151:413–20, 1994.

2. Wortis J and Stone A: The addiction to drug companies. Biol Psychiatry 32:847–9, 1992.

3. Null G: Prozac, Eli Lilly and the FDA. Townsend Lett #115/116: 134, 178–87, 1993.

Chapter 8: The Natural Approach to Anxiety

1. Werbach M: Nutritional Influences on Mental Illness: A Sourcebook of Clinical Research. Third Line Press, Tarzana, CA, 1991.

2. Bruce M and Lader M: Caffeine abstention in the management of anxiety disorders. Psychol Med 19:211–4, 1989.

3. Rudin DO: The major psychoses and neuroses as omega-3 essential fatty acid deficiency syndrome: Substrate pellagra. Biol Psychiatry 16:837–50, 1981.

4. Peterson C, Seligman M, and Valliant G: Pessimistic explanatory style as a risk factor for physical illness: A 35-year longitudinal study. J Person Soc Psych 55:23–7, 1988.

5. Peterson C: Explanatory style as a risk factor for illness. Cog Ther and Res 12:117–30, 1988.

Chapter 9: Natural Alternatives to Anti-Anxiety Drugs

1. Lebot V, Merlin M, and Lindstrom L: Kava: The Pacifc Drug. Yale University Press, New Haven, CT, 1992.

2. Singh Y: Kava: An overview. J Ethnopharmacol 37:13–45, 1992.

3. Meyer HJ: Pharmacology of Kava. In: Ethnopharmacological Search for Psychoactive Drugs. Holmstedt B and Kline NS (eds.). Raven Press, New York, 1979, pp. 133–40.

4. Davies LP, et al.: Kava pyrones and resin: Studies on GABAa, GABAb and benzodiazepine binding sites in rodent brain. Pharm Toxicol 71:120–6, 1992.

5. Holm E, et al.: Studies on the profile of the neurophysiological effects of D,L-kavain: Cerebral sites of action and sleep-wakefulness-rhythm in animals. Arzneim-Forsch 41:673–83, 1991.

6. Jamieson DD and Duffield PH: The antinociceptive action of kava components in mice. Clin Exp Pharmacol Physiol 17:495–508, 1990.

7. Duffield PH and Jamieson D: Development of tolerance to kava in mice. Clin Exp Pharmacol Physiol 18:571–8, 1991.

8. Backhauss and Krieglstein J: Extract of kava (*Piper methysticum*) and its methysticum constituents protect brain tissue against ischemic damage in rodents. Eur J Pharmacol 215:265–9, 1992.

9. Scholing WE and Clausen HD: On the effect of d,l-kavain: Experience with neuronika. Med Klin 72:1301–6, 1977.

10. Lindenberg D and Pitule-Schodel H: D,L-kavain in comparison with oxazepam in anxiety disorders: A double-blind study of clinical effectiveness. Forschr Med 108:49–50, 53–4, 1990.

11. Keledjian J, et al.: Uptake into mouse brain of four compounds present in the psychoactive beverage kava. J Pharm Sci 77: 1003–6, 1988.

12. Kinzler E, Kromer J, and Lehmann E: Clinical efficacy of a kava extract in patients with anxiety syndrome: Double-blind placebo-controlled study over four weeks. Arzneim-Forsch 41:584–8, 1991.

13. Warnecke G: Neurovegetative dystonia in the female climacteric: Studies on the clinical efficacy and tolerance of kava extract WS 1490. Fortschr Med 109:120–2, 1991.

14. Herberg KW: The influence of kava-special extract WS 1490 on safety-relevant performance alone and in combination with ethyl-alcohol. Blutalkohol 30:96–105, 1993.

15. Munte TF, et al.: Effects of oxazepam and an extract of kava roots (*Piper methysticum*) on event-related potentials in a word recognition task. Neuropsychobiol 27:46–53, 1993.

16. Norton SA and Ruze P: Kava dermopathy. J Am Acad Dermatol 31:89–97, 1994.

17. Ruze P: Kava-induced dermopathy: A niacin deficiency. Lancet 335:1442–5, 1990.

18. Mathews JD, et al.: Effects of the heavy usage of kava on physical health: Summary of a pilot survey in an Aboriginal community. Med J Aust 148:548–55, 1988.

19. Heulluy B: Random trial of L.72 with diazepam in cases of nervous depression. Center for Therapeutic Research and Documentation, Paris, France, January 1985.

20. Braverman E and Pfieffer C: The Healing Nutrients Within: Facts, Findings and New Research on Amino Acids. Keats Publishing, New Canaan, CT, 1987.

21. Mulder H and Zoller M: Antidepressive effects of a hypericum extract standardized to the active hypericine content. Arzneim-Forsch 34:918–29, 1984.

22. Woelk H: Multicentric practice-study analyzing the functional capacity in depressive patients. Presented at the 4th International Congress on Phytotherapy, Munich, Germany, September 10–13, 1992, abstract SL54.

Sommer H. Improvement of psychovegetative complaints by hypericum. Presented at the 4th International Congress on Phytotherapy, Munich, Germany, September 10–13, 1992, abstract SL55.

Chapter 10: The Natural Approach to Insomnia

1. Irving A and Jones W: Methods for testing impairment of driving due to drugs. Eur J Clin Pharmacol 43:61–6, 1992.

2. Leathwood P, et al.: Aqueous extract of valerian root (*Valeriana officinalis L.*) improves sleep quality in man. Pharmacol Biochem Beh 17:65–71, 1982.

3. Leathwood PD and Chauffard F: Aqueous extract of valerian reduces latency to fall asleep in man. Planta Medica 54:144–8, 1985.

4. Lindahl O and Lindwall L: Double-blind study of a valerian preparation. Pharmacol Biochem Beh 32:1065–6, 1989.

5. Griffiths W, et al.: Tryptophan and sleep in young adults. Psychophysiol 9:345–56, 1972.

6. Wyatt R, et al.: Effects of L-tryptophan (a natural sedative) on human sleep. Lancet ii:842–6, 1970.

7. Hartman E: L-tryptophan: A rational hypnotic with clinical potential. Am J Psychiatry 134:366–70, 1977.

8. Roufs JB: Review of l-tryptophan and eosinophilia-myalgia syndrome. J Am Diet Assoc 92:844–50, 1992.

9. Caston JC, Roufs JB, Forgarty CM, et al.: Treatment of refractory eosinophilia-myalgia syndrome associated with the ingestion of l-tryptophan containing products. Adv Ther 7:206–28, 1990.

10. Botez M, et al.: Neurologic disorders responsive to folic acid therapy. Can Med Assoc J 115:217–23, 1976.

11. O'Keeffe ST, Gaavin K, and Lavan JN: Iron status and restless legs syndrome in the elderly. Age Ageing 23:200–3, 1994.

Index